menopause
and ADHD

menopause and ADHD

How to navigate hormone flux and neurodivergence

Dr Helen Wall

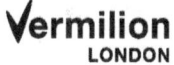

Vermilion
LONDON

VERMILION

UK | USA | Canada | Ireland | Australia
India | New Zealand | South Africa

Vermilion is part of the Penguin Random House group of companies
whose addresses can be found at global.penguinrandomhouse.com

Penguin Random House UK
One Embassy Gardens, 8 Viaduct Gardens, London SW11 7BW

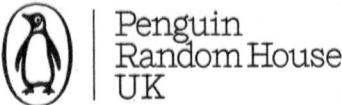

Penguin
Random House
UK

penguin.co.uk

First published by Vermilion in 2026

1

Set in 11.1/14.2pt Calluna
Typeset by Six Red Marbles UK, Thetford, Norfolk

Printed and bound in Great Britain by Clays Ltd, Elcograf S.p.A.

The authorised representative in the EEA is Penguin Random House Ireland,
Morrison Chambers, 32 Nassau Street, Dublin D02 YH68

A CIP catalogue record for this book is available from the British Library

ISBN 9781785046421

Penguin Random House is committed to a sustainable future
for our business, our readers and our planet. This book is made
from Forest Stewardship Council® certified paper.

MIX
Paper | Supporting
responsible forestry
FSC
www.fsc.org   FSC® C018179

To my beautiful daughter, Grace June – may you never have to struggle to be heard or to be seen, and may your voice always be valued in a world that is still learning how to listen to women.

To my loving sons, Ethan and Finlay – may you grow into men who see women fully, who listen without defensiveness, and who stand beside them with respect, courage, and compassion.

May all three of you pursue your own goals in life, whatever they may be, with courage, integrity, and kindness. May you come to know the depth of your own capability.

Finally, to my husband, Jonathan – thank you for your unfaltering support and steadfast love. This work, and I, are stronger because of you.

To women everywhere, let's do this . . .

Contents

Introduction

If you've picked up this book, chances are you've been wondering for a while if there might be more to the way your mind works and why midlife, with all its changes, feels like the hardest part of the journey so far.

Perhaps you've found yourself questioning why strategies that used to hold everything together no longer work. Maybe you've been running on empty, masking the effort it takes just to get through each day, only to find yourself burned out and exhausted. You might be wondering, could this be ADHD? Could perimenopause be making everything worse? Where do you go from here?

In my experience, women who have not been diagnosed with ADHD at a young age often start to have an epiphany around one of two key life stages. The first is when they hit a hormonal stage of flux such as puberty, post-pregnancy or perimenopause. Female hormones are intrinsically linked to how a woman's brain functions (more of this in Chapter 2) and a shift in the stability of this functioning can cause neurodivergence to be unmasked, or, as I like to call it, a period of 'unravelling' to begin. The second peak time is when a mum or a professional identifies possible ADHD in her child and starts to recognise those things in herself as she fits the pieces together. Both occasions are extremely challenging, not least because you already have so much to deal with at these stages of life. Please note that throughout the rest of this book, for conciseness, I will continue to refer to women and girls which, of course, will be inclusive of all those born female, regardless of your current identity.

Despite considerable years at medical school and in training as a junior doctor, I'm sad to say I spent very little time considering the impact of oestrogen and progesterone on the female brain. My day-to-day knowledge of female hormones was centred very much around menstrual disorders, fertility and pregnancy. I've been a doctor for almost 20 years at the time of writing, a GP for over 15 of those, and have worked in various NHS roles for over 25 years. It was not until later in my career, when I began to run a menopause clinic as a registered BMS (British Menopause Society) menopause specialist, that I started to appreciate how perimenopausal women with neurodivergence such as ADHD can be negatively impacted by falling and fluctuating oestrogen and progesterone levels. This observation happened to coincide with both my personal experience of identifying previously unrecognised neurodivergence in my beautiful teenage daughter, and my own perimenopausal journey, in which I felt medically largely unsupported.

The culmination of these life experiences caused me to reflect on an ever-growing catalogue of case studies over the years: those of female patients who had presented, often repeatedly, with burnout, mental health crisis and despair, particularly around puberty, post-childbirth and menopause. This ignited my professional curiosity. One of the things that causes me a great deal of personal distress as a doctor is the recurrent and repeated dismissal of women's lived experiences in healthcare. I am so frustrated that so many of you will have presented your symptoms to a clinician and been diagnosed with anxiety and/or depression. Many of you will now have anxiety and/or depression because of the effects of long-term masking on your mental health. Some of you will sadly have unknowingly self-medicated with substances like alcohol or drugs or tragically burnt out. When the realisation finally hits, many of you describe having masked for so long that you no longer know who you truly are, and a whole new period of trauma unfolds. I will never forget a woman in the prime of her midlife telling me in earnest that society had 'robbed' her of her authentic self. I took it upon myself to encourage her to begin the processing of taking back control, deliberately unmasking and reclaiming that authenticity. However, there's no doubt that this path is a long, rocky road. We will talk a lot more about why the 'mask' often slips in Chapter 2.

It may come as no surprise to you that as I've delved deeper into hormonal effects on women's largely unseen neurodivergence, I've resolved to become part of the solution, not the problem, and so we push on, together. Things are starting to change as more research takes place, but women with ADHD have been and continue to be woefully misunderstood and underrepresented, not least when hormonal flux ensues.

The focus of this book is the menopause, and the symptoms that you may be experiencing which seem to collide and battle with your ADHD to the point that it's negatively impacting your life. I'm here to provide you with not just the toolkit but the validation you need to find strategies to overcome the challenges, reach your ultimate potential and thrive in this period of your life. You're about to learn so much about yourself and understand how to make the best of your health and wellbeing, with conscious choices and awareness. Most of all, **you are always believed here**.

Why masking often fails in midlife

Does ADHD *begin* in perimenopause and menopause? No, but it can certainly become more obvious as the brain becomes overwhelmed, the chemical messengers become less effective or available and the mask that a woman has knowingly or unknowingly used all her life starts to slip. In some women this is not just a slip, it's a complete landslide.

The mask you may wear as a woman with ADHD can slip at any time under challenging circumstances, but there are some key times that this appears more likely to occur. Hormonal shifts, particularly the effects of falling or fluctuating oestrogen levels on key brain receptors and chemical messengers such as dopamine, can play a huge part in stages of life such as puberty, post-pregnancy and perimenopause. We explore more about the effects of hormones on the female brain in Chapter 4, which discusses how your sex hormones impact your brain and how this is so poorly thought about in most day-to-day medical practice.

Midlife can produce an almost perfect storm for the mask to slip. Maybe you have teenagers at home, ageing parents to care for and are facing all the challenges these caring roles can bring. You may be reaching the peak of your career and be tasked with enormous pressure and responsibility or having a moment of reckoning as to what your life is all about. Romantic relationships may be questioned, ended or begun and, like most women over 40, you may start to discover a newfound sense of self that places less importance on pleasing others. Many of the women I speak to describe this mask slipping – and the subsequent implosion of their lives – as 'unravelling' and it can come hard and fast. I have also seen the correlation between many women who have fought long and hard to get their children assessed as neurodivergent suddenly unravelling as they identify these traits in themselves. Your ADHD mask does not slip because you have failed; it slips because it was unsustainable in the first place. You need to understand this and be shown compassion, but more importantly you need to be supported and accepted so you can have compassion for yourself. My hope is that this book will empower you to believe in yourself, your abilities and capabilities. We will talk through all the challenges you may have faced or continue to face as a woman with ADHD in perimenopause (whether diagnosed or not) and provide you with simple and effective tools to advocate for yourself, find balance and regain control.

Throughout the course of this book, I will challenge societal negativity towards neurodivergence. By its very definition, being neurodivergent is not right or wrong; it is different, and different can be super. I will focus on the specific challenges you may face living through your menopause with ADHD because sadly, I've seen too many women in this situation turn up to my GP room in burnout and desperation, undiagnosed and unsupported – and the time for change is now.

Perimenopause and menopause unmask ADHD as a direct result of oestrogen levels fluctuating and falling, which we will explore in depth throughout Chapter 4. This disruption to the status quo overwhelms long-established coping mechanisms that you may not even have been aware of. Perimenopause may be the first time you realise you can no longer rely on your usual strategies to stay afloat. This may have led you to research and resonate with ADHD descriptions, prompting the self-reflection which is so common for so many women during this stage of life.

Many of the symptoms you may present with are often normalised or put down to your hormones alone. Women are often subject to gendered assumptions, such as being more likely to be 'just' tired, anxious or stressed. We need to shout loud and clear that ADHD is lifelong, but as a woman you are more likely to present in midlife having compensated for a long time. Misdiagnosis is rife. Traditional ADHD checklists are prone to missing internalised or masked symptoms – in fact, they are prone to missing women altogether. If a woman has treatment-resistant depression and/or anxiety, we should be looking for a root cause; ADHD and other neurodivergence can be a key one during midlife.

I can't change this overnight, but we can empower each other to be aware and equipped. I hope one day someone reading this book will think 'wow, I can't believe how bad this used to be for women'. I will not tire of telling you that you aren't broken, it is only your scaffolding that likely needs rebuilding. Understanding the interplay of cognition, sensory overlay, sleep, mood, attention and overwhelm allows for better support, more targeted treatments and, most importantly, greater self-compassion and validation. Diagnosis or self-identification is not an endpoint; it's a new beginning. It's the beginning of getting to know and accept yourself in a neuro-typical world that can now start to learn to fit around you rather than the other way around. When we do this for each other as women, we do this for all the women yet to get here.

You are not alone

This book is here to be your companion, your guide, and your supportive hand. Together, we'll explore what it means to unmask in midlife, how ADHD and perimenopause interact, and why fluctuating hormones and burnout so often become the breaking point that finally makes us seek answers. Along the way, you'll learn about pathways to diagnosis, self-acceptance, understanding and self-identification, how to talk to the people around you, and, most importantly, how to find support that feels right for you.

Above all, I hope this book will empower you to know that not only do you need answers, understanding and acceptance, you *deserve* them. Together we can play a small part in ensuring that our daughters, granddaughters and all the women beyond us no longer need to fight to be seen and heard.

How to use this book

I understand that focus, memory and energy can feel in short supply right now. That's why I've designed this book to be flexible and easy to use. Some of the key concepts may be repeated at key points, because 1 understand your current memory troubles may make important concepts harder to follow. If this happens, 1 will also guide you back to where you can read more about these concepts, if you choose to. You can read it cover to cover, or you can dip in and out, depending on what you need most in the moment. There's no 'right way' to read this book – your journey is your own.

- At the start of each chapter, you'll find a bullet-point preview and a short opening paragraph that gives you the gist of what will be covered.
- At the end of each chapter, you'll find a 'TL;DR' (Too Long; Didn't Read) summary to capture the key points without overwhelm.
- Toolkits and resources are highlighted and easy to find, so you can return to them whenever you need practical help.

Why now?

You don't have to struggle in silence. This is a time to uncover, to understand, and to reclaim your energy and confidence. Diagnosis (formal or self-recognised), unmasking and recovery from burnout are not just about survival: they're about empowerment.

You are always believed here. The time is now. And I'm so glad you're here.

Chapter 1
The Many Faces of Neurodivergence

Topics covered in this chapter:

- What is neurodivergence?
- Having ADHD or autism: how it can affect executive function, sensory sensitivity and overlap
- How ADHD often presents differently in women, and the ways women mask
- Could I have ADHD? Screening tools and red flags
- What to do if you suspect undiagnosed ADHD

What is neurodivergence?

As a GP advocating for those with ADHD, one of the most common questions I get asked is 'don't you think we are all a bit on the spectrum?' I have worked with patients within the NHS for almost 25 years, and I can say with absolute certainty that there is no 'normal' and yes, we are all different in how we think, process and navigate the world around us.

This is *neurodiversity*, a concept that recognises how differently our individual brains function and that no two brains are the same. Some of this is genetics, much of it is environment – but being neurodivergent is not just having a few quirks. It is a tangible set of differences in how the brain functions when compared to what is considered typical – or more specifically, neurotypical. I say tangible because we do have evidence from neuroimaging studies, post-mortems and neurophysiological research demonstrating differences in the structure, function, neurochemical transmission (messaging) and brain activity patterns in many people who are neurodivergent compared to those who are neurotypical (more on this in Chapter 2).

The other question sceptics – and sadly these can include colleagues – like to ask me, particularly in relation to ADHD, is 'is it a real thing?' Of course, human nature dictates that some people struggle with biological differences, and it's often harder for them to accept diagnoses for things that haven't got a definitive test. Very rarely has anyone ever questioned me over the authenticity of diabetes or anaemia.

There is very clear evidence that neurodivergence has high heritability, especially in the case of autism (80–90 per cent heritable) and ADHD (70–80 per cent heritable), making these conditions potentially even more heritable than a person's height. There is no single 'neurodivergent gene' – these conditions are instead known as polygenic: caused by the combined effect of several genetic variants (gene differences).

ADHD is also recognised globally and is listed in the DSM-5-TR and ICD-11 as a psychiatric condition. These are the gold-standard diagnostic pathways for diagnosis of mental health conditions used worldwide. DSM-5-TR stands for the fifth edition of the *Diagnostic and Statistical Manual of Mental Disorders*. It is published by the American Psychiatric Association and used globally, both to describe symptoms and criteria for a diagnosis and to help guide management. The fact that ADHD is classified under a catalogue of mental disorders can be upsetting for some but let me reassure you that this system groups ADHD under a set of conditions called 'neurodevelopmental disorders'. These conditions affect how the brain develops, functions or processes information, which in my view is testament to the fact that ADHD is not a set of behavioural or character flaws; it is instead a recognised pattern of traits related to a developmental difference in how the brain is wired. ADHD is not a mental illness but – a neurodevelopmental difference, and as we will explore, it comes with many evolutionary benefits.

Similarly, ICD-11 stands for International Classification of Diseases; 11th Revision and is published by the World Health Organization (WHO). Its scope is much broader, covering a whole magnitude of conditions. Again, it is used globally and across the breadth of medicine for diagnostic criteria, statistics and public health planning.

Neurodivergence, put simply, refers to a brain that functions and processes things differently from the typical way we might expect (or to those who are neurotypical). You could argue that what we come to expect is largely down to us as a society and is not 'black and white'. Neurodivergence is not a medical term (nor a diagnosis) but it is used as an umbrella term for a range of presentations including ADHD, autistic spectrum disorder (ASD), dyslexia, dyspraxia and dyscalculia. It is not uncommon for someone to have several of these in combination (and not surprising, given their heritable nature). It is also important to say from the outset that neurodivergence is a difference, not a deficit. I truly believe that having a neurodivergent brain is not an automatic barrier to living a hugely successful and happy life; making those who are neurodivergent live in a society made solely for the neurotypical brain can, however, be a significant challenge. Some of the most resilient, determined and successful people I've met have been very clearly neurodivergent. The key is to recognise when you or someone else is neurodivergent, celebrate the amazing qualities (of which there are many) and create an environment that enables success. I hope this book helps more people to do just that.

Having ADHD or autism: how it can affect executive function, sensory sensitivity and overlap

While there are key differences between those with ADHD and autistic people, there is also significant overlap. One of the key challenges if you are autistic or have ADHD is the significant difference in your brain's executive function. Think of this as the brain's management centre, responsible for **planning, organising, starting, finishing, shifting between tasks, working memory** and **regulating emotions**. This difference in executive function can show up in many ways, including time blindness (not recognising how much time you do or don't have, often leading to lateness), procrastination and constantly losing belongings. You may find you often struggle to plan and execute a given task in a logical order; the necessary steps may not be obvious to you, or you might lose focus midway through, no matter how much effort you put in. You likely struggle with emotional dysregulation leading to a rapid change in your mood and impulsivity in your reactions. You can often react in haste and reflect later.

The ADHD brain differs in how it regulates dopamine activity (as well as other chemical messengers which we will discuss in Chapter 2), meaning you often seek out dopamine-activating events or activities which can vary massively in their benefits and downsides. For example, some people may take up exercise, learn a new hobby or find a creative outlet while others may turn to gambling, excessive spending or overeating high-fat, sugary foods to get that boost. Some may even seek dopamine in more subtle ways, such as by creating an argument. In autistic people this differing executive brain function may show up as being fixated on the planning of a task but struggling to get started on any given plan, relying heavily on routine and structure, and difficulty shifting attention. If you are autistic, you may also become overwhelmed and have delayed or intense emotional responses, often linked to sensory or information overload.

If you have ADHD and/or are autistic, you will likely have some degree of sensory sensitivity. This means you may experience sensory inputs from touch, sound, light, smell, taste and temperature more (or, in rarer cases, less) intensely than your neurotypical peers. While sensory processing differences are a core diagnostic feature of autism, with 80–95 per cent of autistic people affected, they may also be experienced by 40–60 per cent of people with ADHD. This can manifest as overwhelm in crowded, noisy environments, irritability with the way clothes feel against the skin and an aversion to or seeking out strong tastes or smells. With ADHD, you may express sensory sensitivity as constant fidgeting, moving or chewing rather than verbalising your discomfort. This can also be referred to as 'stimming'.

Many autistic people also have ADHD (and vice versa), often identified in neurodivergent communities as AuDHD. Some studies suggest this overlap can occur in 20–50 per cent of individuals. Despite this statistic, AuDHD is not yet recognised as a separate diagnosis in the diagnostic manual DSM-5-TR. Autistic spectrum disorder (ASD) and ADHD are listed as separate conditions that can co-occur.

We'll come back to this topic in Chapter 7, when I discuss how tricky it is to get a holistic assessment of ADHD through the lens of perimenopause – currently, it's also almost impossible for a GP to refer a patient for an assessment that will take a holistic overview of that patient for all possible neurodivergent traits and their coexistence. That's why I hope to arm you with the information in this book, to ensure that you can navigate this situation as effectively as possible. While there is significant overlap in many of the traits between the two conditions, they can also clash in their needs. For example, ADHD thrives on novelty and autism thrives on routine, meaning living with both can be even more of a challenge that adds to ultimate burnout in perimenopause and beyond.

While both the sensory sensitivity and executive function differences of ADHD and autistic people are often seen as disadvantages, I feel strongly that with the right understanding and environment they can be significantly advantageous. In fact, there are several theories that suggest that such differences may have developed as evolutional advantages in certain populations. For example, some ADHD traits may have been beneficial in hunter-gatherer societies, where being able to quickly shift focus, be intuitive to danger, hyperfocus and maintain high energy levels to act quickly and changeably may have conferred significant survival advantages on those individuals.

Your ADHD and/or autistic brain will have a raft of positive traits born from your sensory sensitivity and executive function even today. Being finely tuned into your sensory inputs often manifests as heightened perception and intuition: the ability to pick up on subtle sounds, textures, light and patterns. This sensory fine-tuning can also extend to emotional intelligence and, even if you struggle to express it, you are often very perceptive to others' non-verbal cues and have strong empathic ability. You may be very creative and excel in jobs that lend themselves to free thought, innovation and artistic flair. Executive function differences can lead to 'outside the box' thinking and free-flowing ideas. If you are autistic or have ADHD, you likely become hyper focused on things that interest you and can be extremely productive and masterful in any such given task or skill. With ADHD you often bring high energy and an engaging passion, while autistic people often act from a core sense of what is right and logical. These traits can make for passionate advocates and strong engaging leaders in the right fields.

How ADHD often presents differently in women, and the ways women mask

Like many things in medicine, ADHD has been viewed with a male gaze for a long time. Diagnostic criteria across the world are linked to how boys and men present, and this has shaped what people, including those in the education and healthcare systems, recognise as ADHD. This is especially noticeable in ADHD where I've heard many parents of girls and young women frustratedly recount how they've been told time and time again that their daughters cannot possibly have ADHD as they are not in the least bit disruptive. In fact, they've often been highlighted as model pupils, perfectionists with a real desire to please. You may well be one of these women or girls. Similarly, I've met a huge number of women who have been told that their successful career or ability to succeed in whatever guise means they can't possibly have ADHD.

If this is all sounding familiar, then I'm sorry. What absolute nonsense. The truth is that those born female often present very differently with ADHD to those born male, meaning women like you have often gone undiagnosed and unsupported for years. Girls and women often internalise their symptoms and behaviours to fit in, something known as **masking**. This is often an unconscious act. Rather than being disruptive through poor behaviour, women with ADHD are often so keen to please and to fit in that they become perfectionist, to the detriment of their own emotional and mental wellbeing. They do this for years until they become exhausted and eventually burn out.

There are several ways girls and women may mask their ADHD difficulties. Here are some of the ways you may have done or continue to do just this . . .

Overcompensation through perfectionism

You may work extremely hard to put on a front of being organised and tidy. Your desk or workspace may be immaculate and your personal appearance the same. You may spend an inordinate amount of time prepping and double-checking things you must deliver at school, work or socially. You may feel a constant worry you will forget something, make a mistake or get things wrong, and ruminate on how that can be avoided. Back home in safety, you may exist in total chaos and express overwhelm with frequent meltdowns among loved ones in a safe space.

Excessive people pleasing

Women and girls who are masking ADHD will often say 'yes' to things as a matter of routine. You may wish to avoid confrontation and mask your perceived inadequacies. By saying yes, you can feel able and likeable. You may constantly read the room with a heightened sense of intuition and adjust your interactions accordingly to fit in. Likewise, you may feel the need to apologise on repeat and try containing your inner restlessness to avoid seeming 'too much'. You may overthink what others think of you and rerun conversations and interactions internally on repeat. As a result, inner turmoil may now seem like a normal state of being for you.

Mimicking to blend in

Many women and girls with ADHD may learn through experience to blend in socially. You may do this by internally scripting interactions or rehearsing expected conversations.

This may also manifest as copying the way others speak, facial expressions or body language to not stand out too much. You may express learned social behaviours that never truly feel like you are expressing your true self.

Hiding executive function challenges

Women and girls with ADHD may over-prepare to ensure things at least seem under control and that their forgetfulness and challenges with working memory aren't noticeable. You may spend a large amount of time writing lists, keeping diaries and notebooks, using sticky notes and apps to try and stay on track. Tasks can take much longer but this is unlikely to be obvious to most other people outside of the home. If this mask slips, females are often labelled by society as scatty or ditzy, reinforcing the need to hide difficulties and, unsurprisingly, potentially further affecting self-esteem.

Supressing emotions outside of safe spaces

You may try and hide your emotional dysregulation for fear of being seen as oversensitive or dramatic. You may often have a strong and overwhelming response to perceived rejection (rejection sensitive dysphoria) and can mask this by pretending not to care at all. This can manifest as aloofness or calm on the outside while inner emotional chaos rages. Your loved ones may bear the brunt when this inevitably needs an outlet. If this is not understood and managed by loved ones, relationships will suffer and disintegrate repeatedly over time.

Internalising hyperactivity and impulsivity

Women will often go to great lengths not to be disruptive to others in a social or group setting. Culturally, women are seen to be productive homemakers and multitaskers. You will likely take steps to internalise your restlessness or turn it into acceptable productivity like cleaning or errands. Mental over-activity and restlessness are often manifested as overthinking, self-criticism and an inability to 'switch off'. You may some-times prefer to silence yourself and not engage at all to limit the chances of interrupting others by blurting out or saying something inappropriate.

Most of us will be exhausted just by reading the above descriptions of the ways women may mask. This may be your reality day in, day out just to survive – and consequently, you may be on an understandable and inevitable path to burnout. If this is you, you will likely recognise these things in yourself and suddenly understand why you constantly feel so tired. Masking may have helped you succeed at school, socially and in the workplace but it has also come at the cost of exhaustion, burnout, low self-esteem and, likely, a delayed diagnosis.

How can you not know you are masking? Meet Janice

Some may find this notion hard to countenance. How could someone not realise all their lives they are literally struggling to 'think straight'? Let me explain by telling you about Janice. Janice, as far as anyone knew, did not have ADHD, but she did have a disability that remained hidden for many years. By telling her story, I would like to demonstrate the parallels of how your own ADHD can remain hidden for so many years – even from yourself.

Janice was born many years ago with two healthy-looking eyes; however, one of them was undiagnosed blind since birth. No one – not even Janice – knew that one of her eyes did not work. This way of seeing (medically known as monocular vision) was entirely normal to Janice, even though she spent a large part of her life sensing she wasn't quite as easily able as everyone else. She felt different but didn't know why, so she pushed on. Janice changed how she did things to cope, most of the time subconsciously and without fuss. These changes were often subtle; a slight head or full eye turn, brighter lights and colours, placing her hand down before a cup as a reference point for lack of depth perception.

Janice had learned to 'mask' her disability and cope with one eye, even though she never really knew this was the case. At times she felt frustrated, upset and incapable, and at times others thought the same but she pushed on and developed great resilience and skill. One day she sustained an injury to her good eye and became completely blind. Suddenly all the battling she had done and all the coping mechanisms she put in place no longer helped. People around Janice couldn't understand why she had gone from fine to completely blind due to an injury affecting just one eye. Despite having demonstrated the most amazing resilience and grit her whole life for getting this far with one healthy eye, Janice felt like she'd failed because suddenly she couldn't do all the things she had previously managed to do. Despite never asking for accommodations or help before, she felt guilty and shameful having to ask now.

Most women do this their whole lives to compensate for their ADHD; they may not even have been aware of this for most of it. The hormonal impact can be a step too far (like losing the sight in your one good eye) and the coping mechanisms that have kept you afloat for so long are no longer able to do so. I call this unravelling, and I know so many of you relate to that term. The reality is it isn't ludicrous for women to get to midlife and suddenly realise they may have ADHD (or any other neurodivergence). What is ludicrous is that firstly, we have not helped them recognise this sooner and secondly, we question them for recognising it now.

Could I have ADHD? Screening tools and red flags

If you haven't yet got an ADHD diagnosis but think you may have it, you may wish to screen yourself as a first step. We will revisit this in Chapter 5 where I explain how to take a positive screen to your GP and other things you can do to try and get some support. The ASRS vi.i (Adult ADHD Self-Report Scale Part A) is a screening questionnaire, developed by the World Health Organization (WHO) and used by GPs and other clinicians as a first step in any queried ADHD presentation. The good news is it is widely and freely available online and you can find this on ADHD UK's website (see the 'Resources' section at the end of the book).

This short form asks six questions to assess inattention (difficult starting/completing tasks) and hyperactivity and impulsivity (e.g. being fidgety and restless). A score of four or more positive answers in Part A suggests further evaluation may be warranted. This is of course a very crude measure without much detail or context at all, but it is a widely used and an easy starting point. There are several other ADHD scales available online that tend to be used by specialists to aid in the diagnostic process, such as the Conners' Adult ADHD Rating Scales (CAARS) and the Wender Utah Rating Scale (WURS). The irony is never lost on me that these forms require concentration, focus and completion, all of which can be challenging for those affected by ADHD. Nevertheless, many ADHD clinics request such forms as part of the referral and diagnostic process. If you are struggling to complete said forms, forgetting, procrastinating or can't focus, I'd recommend asking a loved one for help. Be kind to yourself; most people I refer for an ADHD assessment feel the same way.

For those of you still unsure, here are some key traits that may indicate ADHD in women (formal diagnostic criteria can be found in Chapter 5):

Inattention Signs

- Chronic forgetfulness (keys, appointments, conversations, passwords)
- Frequently losing possessions (often things you've just had hold of and put down)
- Trouble sustaining focus in conversations, meetings, or when reading
- Easily distracted by unrelated thoughts or stimuli mid-task
- Disorganisation, poor time management, inability to plan time e.g. believing you have more time than you do to get ready then panicking at the last minute
- Difficulty starting, planning and completing tasks in a logical and succinct manner, as well as difficulty staying on task
- Procrastination despite knowing and fearing the consequences of not starting or completing a task

Hyperactivity-Impulsivity Signs

- Restlessness (feeling internally agitated; overthinking; can't switch off thoughts even if not physically fidgety)
- Interrupting others, blurting out responses
- Difficulty waiting in queues or through long conversations; impatient
- Taking on multiple tasks and abandoning them midway through

- Impulsive spending or decision-making; inability to plan for the long term
- Having only two time zones: now and not now

Red flags signalling undiagnosed ADHD in women

- Chronic forgetfulness, disorganisation, procrastination, chronic exhaustion, overwhelm
- Restlessness (mental and/or physical), impulsive decisions, sudden mood shifts
- Difficulty with focus, time management, emotional regulation
- Rejection sensitivity, frequent burnout, internal chaos despite external control
- Co-existing anxiety or depression, often misdiagnosed or misunderstood, or not responding to repeated treatment

What to do if you suspect undiagnosed ADHD

If you suspect you may have ADHD, here's a checklist of what to do. Firstly, complete the ASRS screening questionnaire. Having a positive score does not mean you have ADHD, but it is a positive indicator. Next, if you haven't already, confide in someone you trust about your concerns. I would also encourage you to think about what a formal diagnosis may feel like or change within your life. For some it can be incredibly validating to have an answer for the years of feeling different and exhausted. For others it can feel unnecessary and debilitating. For many it can be an extremely emotional time with conflicting and rapidly changing or simultaneous feelings of loss, anger, guilt and sadness, especially if the diagnosis has come later in life. In Chapter 6, we will go into detail about the pros and cons of seeking a diagnosis in midlife and how self-identification may be another option for you.

You do not need a formal diagnosis to start to rebuild your life and get support. While medication for ADHD can be helpful to some, it isn't the only path to support. Chapter 7 takes an in-depth look at not just ADHD medication, but also HRT and the potential interplay between the two. If you self-identify as having ADHD, you can still access a wealth of online resources, groups and support networks to improve your wellbeing.

If you do want to seek a diagnosis, it is important to consider your symptoms across the course of your whole life and its various settings (school, work, home). It may be helpful to speak to others around you, such as siblings, parents and lifelong friends. Sometimes people have access to old school reports which may offer insights into their academic performance and behaviour as children (remembering that how girls present in the classroom is often very different to boys).

We don't think ADHD develops in adulthood (emerging studies may disagree) but we know it often goes unrecognised in childhood and sadly, many years beyond that in women. I would also recommend that you identify why and how these traits of ADHD affect you on a day-to-day basis. For women, this may not be overtly obvious to others and may need spelling out. Writing this down can be helpful for all parties.

I've lost count of the number of women who have reached out to me online to tell me how much anxiety the thought of taking this suspicion to their GP causes them. Each time I hear this, I feel incredibly sad because no one – man or woman, child or adult – should feel this way about seeing their GP. However, I also recognise that this recurrent fear and anxiety comes from a real place of experiencing dismissal by some GPs. Many women have masked and fought their whole lives to survive with all the ADHD traits and fears of criticism and rejection I've highlighted, and to be dismissed at this juncture has a significantly negative impact on their wellbeing. To help you prepare, do your research, make notes of your traits and their effects, go to your GP open-minded (demanding a referral and being angry, while understandable, won't help). It may help to take a loved one for support if you can, and to have handwritten notes with you. These notes can include a comprehensive history (e.g. things that happened in childhood that could be relevant) compiled with the help of your loved ones, if you think you may struggle to express everything during the consultation.

This first chapter has been an overview of neurodivergence, specifically ADHD and how you may have masked all your life. We will revisit masking in more depth along with overwhelm, the effects of hormones and everything in between as we traverse through the chapters that follow. Similarly, we will revisit taking your concerns to your GP in more depth in Chapter 5 because I know that this can be extremely challenging and anxiety provoking for many. As a GP, I wanted to mention this early on because it is one of the commonest questions I receive and I'm sad (but understanding) at how much anxiety it causes. I do not believe any GP wants a patient to feel this way, but a lack of awareness, knowledge and timely solutions can inevitably lead to this outcome. My aim is to empower you to hold your ground, know that you are not alone, not in the wrong and deserve – at the very least – to be heard.

Things you could say to say your GP (when worried you have ADHD)

What do you want?

- 'I'd like to talk today about the possibility that I might have ADHD' (be clear, concise and direct)

- 'I've been reading about ADHD in adult women and a lot of what I've read fits me' (show you've thought about it)
- 'I'm struggling with a lot of symptoms that are affecting my day-to-day life and I'd like to discuss an assessment for ADHD' (shows the impact and a clear request)

How has it affected you?

- 'I've always found x, y, z hard since childhood' (links back through the years)
- 'The same issues have affected me in my relationships, work, home life by x, y, z' (explains transition of affects through life)

How is it affecting you now?

- 'I no longer feel I can cope like I used to and it's causing x, y, z' (brings the focus to your current day-to-day life)
- 'I think I have masked all my life, and this is evidenced through x, y, z' (shows why you may seem effective to others)

What has masking taken from you or what does it continue to take?

- 'Despite looking in control, I constantly feel overwhelmed, guilty and incapable' (explains how masking makes you feel)
- 'I feel worn out and exhausted just keeping on top of life' (as above)

Why do you want an assessment?

- 'I want to explore a diagnosis to feel like I can finally understand why my life has felt so hard' (gives the

GP an understanding of how important assessment is to you)
- 'I want to be assessed so I can access medication and/or support at work' (gives tangible, practical reasoning for being assessed)

TL;DR – Chapter 1: The Many Faces of Neurodivergence

- Neurodivergence is brain function that differs from the typical (neurotypical) pattern in real, measurable differences in brain structure, chemistry and function.
- It includes conditions like ADHD, autism, dyslexia, dyspraxia and dyscalculia.
- Neurodivergent conditions are thought to be highly heritable: ADHD (70–80 per cent), autism (80–90 per cent).
- ADHD and autism are officially recognised in the gold-standard diagnostic pathways DSM-5-TR and ICD-11.

Key traits of neurodivergent brains

- Differences in executive function are common (difficulty planning, organising, managing emotions).
- Sensory sensitivity to light, sound, touch, etc. affects many with ADHD/autism.
- These differences are often seen as disadvantages but can be strengths (creativity, intuition, hyperfocus).

ADHD in women: misrepresented and misdiagnosed

- Diagnostic models have a male bias; girls and women often go undiagnosed.
- Many women mask symptoms to fit in: people-pleasing, perfectionism, scripting social interactions.
- They often present as perfectionists, high functioning and internally suffering from anxiety, depression or burnout.
- Masking leads to exhaustion, identity confusion and late diagnoses.

How undiagnosed ADHD can show up in women

- Chronic forgetfulness, disorganisation, procrastination
- Restlessness (mental and/or physical), impulsive decisions
- Difficulty with focus, time management, emotional regulation
- Rejection sensitivity (see page 64), frequent burnout, internal chaos despite external control
- Co-existing anxiety or depression, often misdiagnosed or misunderstood, low self-esteem

What to do if you suspect you have ADHD

- Start with the ASRS v1.1 screening tool (freely available online, see Resources).
- Consider how traits have affected you across your life and environments.

- Confide in someone you trust and prepare to speak to your GP.
- You don't need a diagnosis to access help, strategies or support.

Tips for speaking to your GP

✓ Be clear and concise about what you need, want and expect: 'I want to talk about the possibility I have ADHD.'
✓ Link symptoms to lifelong patterns and daily impact.
✓ Explain the emotional toll of masking and burnout.
✓ Bring notes, examples, and even a loved one to support you.
✓ Stay open and prepared; diagnosis and treatment may take time.
✓ Try to be positive and proactive but assertive about your requests and concerns.

Chapter 2
From ADHD Life to Perimenopause and Menopause: What's Going on in My Body and Mind?

Topics covered in this chapter:

- How neurodivergent women manage careers, parenting and life
- Overcompensation, burnout and why masking often fails in midlife
- A medical overview of perimenopause and menopause
- Hormonal shifts and how they impact the brain (including differences in the ADHD brain)
- Common symptoms that overlap with neurodivergence – and how to navigate this

In this chapter we will explore how ADHD may have shaped who you are as you navigated the key aspects of life and arrived at midlife, particularly careers and parenting. We will explore how ADHD and a subconscious or conscious desire to succeed or blend in may have led you to mask all your life, become overwhelmed and burn out. We will look at how the ADHD brain may vary from your neurotypical peers and how this may lead you to chase dopamine, a key chemical messenger in your brain. Then we will look at the medical aspects of perimenopause and menopause, and how the hormonal changes that occur during this life stage can impact your brain both with and without ADHD, leading to unmasking and the quickening of potential burnout. Finally, this chapter aims to empower you to move forward in your journey to seeking the answers and understanding you have needed for so long.

How neurodivergent women manage careers, parenting and life

As we covered in Chapter 1, neurodivergent women can be extremely successful in every aspect of life. However, without recognition of the recurrent challenges you may face and the right support and acceptance this can come at a huge personal cost. Like we discussed, many of you mask your symptoms for decades, especially when outside of the home and away from 'safe spaces'. Outwardly, you often seem to be extremely organised, measured and doing well. You may develop perfectionist traits, going to great lengths to please others and stay in control. Your apparent ability to maintain constant multitasking and high energy levels may be the envy of others around you. The reality is often very different. This way of living is at best exhausting and at worst putting you on the road to burnout and a mental health crisis that will hit you when you least expect it (some of you may be here right now).

As a woman with ADHD, you are most likely very empathic with high intuition and emotional insight. You are often creative and have good problem-solving intelligence. If you find something you are acutely interested in you can be extremely passionate and engaged. Hyperfocus (a key trait of ADHD) used in the right way can be super productive. As well as these special qualities that make you an amazing human, you may also experience key challenges that may get in your way of success and happiness if not managed appropriately. Some of these include executive function differences (difficulty planning, starting or completing tasks, poor working memory), emotional dysregulation, low self-esteem and internalised hyperactivity (never being able to truly rest).

Reaching your true potential will require an understanding of your deeper self and how your brain functions that often only comes with time. You may only now be starting to truly understand how your brain and emotions react, or you may – like many other midlife women – be about to embark on this journey having reached crisis point. This may indeed be the reason you are here reading this book. You may feel bereft of the time you have lost and anxious about how to proceed. This book aims to hold your hand on this journey, whatever point you are at.

Careers

School may have been a tough ride for you, or you may have masked so well you felt you were invincible. The reality is probably somewhere in between but I would hazard a guess that the chances of the education system having picked up your ADHD are slim. Sadly, girls with ADHD remain severely under recognised in our education systems, not least because they are rarely disruptive due to the internalised nature of any hyperactivity and inattention.

Despite this, you may have used your energy and resilience to develop a promising career. There is a frustrating misconception even among medical colleagues that those with ADHD cannot be successful in the workplace. It will not surprise you to know that I completely and vehemently disagree. That said, you will likely do best in the workplace if you understand your strengths and weaknesses and chose a career that plays well to both.

Equally, if an employer and work peers can understand these strengths and weaknesses well and accommodate them, they too can have a super productive, engaging and innovative colleague or employee. The difficulty for women in achieving this state of mutual understanding, of course, is that you are often masking and misunderstood for much of your life. In fact, so many women don't even recognise this in themselves until the mask slips and things unravel. Many women receive such a late diagnosis that they are not supported or enabled to thrive in any setting, let alone their education or career.

Parenting

Parenting is challenging for everyone and some of these challenges can be exacerbated by having ADHD.

Children bring a degree of chaos to any home, from birth to teenage years. The difference in how your brain's executive function plays out with ADHD can exacerbate this challenge and in turn impact your confidence in your parental abilities. Difficulty with planning, task completion, time management and preparation – not just for yourself but another human that you are responsible for – can add a significant layer of overwhelm. If you experience sensory overload with ADHD, you can find the level of noise, mess or repetitive physical touch with young children particularly distressing. The challenge of forming and maintaining routines and ease of distraction may lead to zoning out and seeming disinterested.

It is no coincidence that one of the most common times for women to request an assessment for ADHD or autism is when their child is in the process of being assessed and diagnosed for the same. Suddenly a stark realisation dawns that they too may be undiagnosed as years of struggling and overwhelm flash before them and start to make some sense. Studies suggest that the chance of a parent with ADHD having a child with ADHD is between 25 and 50 per cent. This is much higher than the general population, who have a risk of 5–7 per cent. Parenting children with neurodivergence when you are neurodivergent is a whole new ball game.

All children, but especially those with neurodivergence, need predictable routines and structure to thrive. They may also be more prone to emotional meltdowns and overwhelm, both of which can be harder to manage as a parent trying to navigate differences in executive function and emotional overwhelm of your own. Dysregulation and crisis management can become the daily norm. Seeing your child struggle with things you too have found challenging can be very triggering for adults and this can lead to a time of great stress and ultimate reflection. It has long been said that comparison is the thief of joy and in my experience, there's no shortage of ADHD mums comparing themselves to other mums and often feeling inadequate for it throughout perimenopause and beyond. Reflecting on your years of parenting while dealing with perimenopausal derailment and looking after hormonal teenagers who may also be neurodivergent is tough, and we don't talk about this nearly enough.

Overcompensation, burnout and why masking often fails in midlife

Masking ADHD usually involves overcompensation such as obsessive planning, scripting conversations and overpreparation of meetings or social events. While this may make you more likely to succeed socially and in your career, over time it can lead to chronic stress and burnout. Imposter syndrome is incredibly common if you have ADHD. Despite evidence to the contrary, you may feel fraudulent, unworthy and not capable of your achievements. This is often magnified in women with ADHD; one day you're impressing everyone at work in a meeting, the next you can't find your keys or plan a trip to the supermarket. The inconsistency of your abilities and masking to stay on top of things feeds imposter syndrome.

Success feels like it's based on effort not ability, which understandably feeds an endless stream of self-doubt and exhaustion.

You may be extremely bright but fall short of your ultimate potential due to disorganisation and inconsistent attention and memory. The disconnect between what you are capable of and what you can follow through with consistently fuels self-doubt and ultimately leads to burnout; this can be particularly evident in perimenopause when you are already juggling so many other emotional and physical changes. Perimenopause and menopause are a time of awakening and self-reflection. Who are you? How did you get here, and where do you want to be?

Not only do you behave inconsistently with others, you remain inconsistent and unreliable to yourself which can slowly but surely chip away at your self-esteem. If not supported and accepted in relationships, employment and social settings, this can lead to significant loss and in turn self-loathing. It is no wonder so many women with ADHD also have a coexisting diagnosis of anxiety or depression. So many of the women I meet report being told repeatedly that they are careless, make 'silly' mistakes and are not living up to their potential, which essentially gives them an undeserved sense of laziness and failure. If you have access to your old school reports, I suspect you will see similar comments there. Internalised shame is very real and sadly very common; worst of all, it can be notoriously hard to undo. If you recognise this, please also recognise that you are not alone and you are not a failure. If you are struggling with your inner voice, Chapter 6 provides insight and tools to support you.

Burnout

Burnout with ADHD is a state of not just physical but also mental and emotional exhaustion. If you are affected you may feel extreme fatigue, brain fog and a complete inability to focus, concentrate or acquire any motivation. Burnout often drains your energy, joy and sense of self. Neurodivergent burnout goes deeper. It's not just exhaustion; it's the weight of constantly adapting, masking and surviving in a world that wasn't built with you in mind. Below I've outlined the subtle but significant differences between general burnout and neurodivergent burnout:

General Burnout

- Definition: A state of physical, emotional and mental exhaustion caused by prolonged stress, usually related to work or caregiving.
- Core features (according to WHO):
  - Emotional exhaustion (feeling drained, depleted)
  - Depersonalisation or cynicism (detaching, feeling negative)
  - Reduced sense of accomplishment (feeling ineffective, unproductive)

- Causes: Often linked to workload, lack of control, poor workplace support, or high demands with insufficient recovery time.
- Recovery: Rest, stress reduction, workplace adjustments, time out, therapy, lifestyle changes.

Neurodivergent Burnout

- Definition: A specific type of burnout experienced by autistic, ADHD, or otherwise neurodivergent people. It happens when the cumulative effort of masking, adapting to neurotypical environments, sensory overload and chronic stress exceeds capacity.
- Core features:
  - Heightened exhaustion: deeper and more pervasive than typical burnout, often affecting basic functioning.

- Loss of skills: temporary regression in coping strategies, executive function, speech, or social ability.
- Increased sensitivity: sensory overwhelm, reduced tolerance for stressors.
- Identity impact: distress around authenticity, masking and belonging.

- Causes:
  - Long-term masking (hiding traits to 'fit in')
  - Navigating inaccessible environments (noise, routines, social demands)
  - Lack of accommodations or understanding
- Recovery: Often requires longer recovery periods, reducing or stopping masking, accommodations in environment, self-compassion and community support. Time out alone won't 'fix it'; consistent and extensive structural change is often needed.

Burnout often leads to withdrawal, both socially and within work and family settings. It is a sad situation that women are allowed to get to this point time and time again before anyone identifies they are neurodivergent. Often women in this situation are diagnosed with a mental health disorder such as anxiety or depression and medicated accordingly. While there may be a coexisting condition, this diagnosis doesn't consider the journey to and root causes of burnout.

A medical overview of perimenopause and menopause

The perimenopause is the transitional phase leading up to menopause, the subsequent stage of life when a woman's periods have ceased for 12 months with no other cause identified. The perimenopause can last up to 10 years before periods stop, although it is usually much shorter. During this time, ovarian function starts to decline, leading to fluctuating hormone levels and overall eventual reduction of oestrogen and progesterone.

During perimenopause, periods may be irregular and haphazard in their timings, heavier or lighter in their flow, and longer or shorter in their duration. Continuing to have periods in whatever form does not mean you are not in perimenopause and experiencing all the challenges it presents. Hormonal levels go up and down in perimenopause so measuring them is largely unhelpful for diagnosis. Take follicle stimulating hormone (FSH) for example; put simply, this hormone is released by the pituitary gland in your brain to tell the ovaries to produce an egg every month. When your ovaries start to wind down, the brain eventually releases more FSH to try and get them going again. As such, your FSH level will be high in menopause but in perimenopause it's often normal, at least in the earlier days. For this reason, testing FSH is unhelpful for most women entering perimenopause at the expected time, and certainly isn't diagnostic. The average age of menopause in the UK is around 51 years but there is huge variation in this and it's important we don't assume every issue in midlife is automatically related to perimenopause or menopause. Hot sweats, night sweats, irregular periods, mood changes, brain fog, memory issues, dry skin, fatigue and aches and pains can all be very common in perimenopausal women but so many of these symptoms can also be signs of another condition. I'd encourage you not to assume any cause and seek clarity from a healthcare professional.

The first-line treatment for symptomatic perimenopause and menopause is hormone replacement therapy (HRT), according to all available guidance from NICE NG23; British Menopause Society (BMS); Royal College of Obstetricians and Gynaecologists (RCOG); International Menopause Society (IMS); and North American Menopause Society (NAMS). It would be remiss of me not to highlight that despite the known efficacy of HRT, there are a significant number of women who cannot safely take HRT, choose not to take it or struggle to tolerate it. Unfortunately, there are also significant training gaps in medical education when it comes to midlife women, hormones and their menopause journey.

While all UK GPs should receive some training in basic menopause care, the depth of knowledge can vary hugely. You may be fortunate to have access to a GP or practice clinician who has an interest in this area, has completed extra training and qualifications in menopause care, or has extensive experience of seeing women in menopause, but this is certainly not a given.

As a jobbing GP I can tell you that UK general practice is vast and menopause care is complex. In my experience, no two women are the same and there should be no one-size-fits-all approach. A good menopause assessment will look at you as an individual, with all your quirks and needs, and even then, getting the right fit is often a process of trial and error. The depth of consultation required to do menopausal women justice is in my opinion often too large for a standard NHS GP appoint-ment however well the GP or practice clinician is trained. Below, I provide some guidelines about what you can realistically expect from an NHS GP when it comes to your perimenopause and menopause care and what may require a more specialist approach, such as from a GP who has perhaps taken time out to delve deeper or referral to a specialist menopause clinic.

The basics of menopause care

What you can (and should) realistically expect from your GP

Areas that your GP should be able to discuss with you:

- Recognition of symptoms: hot flushes, night sweats, mood changes, sleep disturbance, urogenital symptoms, irregular/absent periods.

- Diagnosis: usually clinical in women over 45 (no blood tests needed).
- First-line treatment: HRT as the most effective option for vasomotor symptoms.
- Types of HRT: oestrogen-only (for women without a womb) vs combined oestrogen + progesterone (for those with a womb).
- Non-HRT options: lifestyle advice, CBT, and non-hormonal medications (e.g. SSRIs/SNRIs, clonidine).
- Vaginal oestrogen: safe for urogenital symptoms, can be used long-term.
- Risks and benefits: broad understanding that benefits outweigh risks for most women under 60 or within 10 years of menopause.
- Contraception in perimenopause: awareness that pregnancy is still possible until menopause is confirmed.

Areas where GP knowledge and confidence may be patchy (unless they have undertaken further training):

- Newer formulations: understanding of body-identical vs synthetic HRT (e.g. micronised proges-terone vs medroxyprogesterone).
- Dosing nuances: adjusting oestrogen dose/form (gel, patch, spray, tablets) when symptoms persist.
- Testosterone: awareness that it may help low libido, but many GPs aren't confident prescribing it as it's unlicensed and there is limited support for its use.
- Complex patients: women with migraines, clotting disorders, cardiovascular disease, breast cancer history.
- Premature ovarian insufficiency (POI): ensuring diagnosis and long-term HRT for bone/heart protection.

- Non-classic symptoms: joint pains, palpitations, cognitive changes which aren't always recognised as menopausal.
- Long-term HRT safety: detailed risk discussion (e.g. breast cancer risk with different progestogens, stroke risk by age/formulation).
- Stopping/restarting HRT: strategies for weaning, recurrence of symptoms, or trying again later.

Understanding whether HRT is right for you

I still hear from women who have been told they absolutely cannot have HRT, for example from women who experience migraines, when this is not the case providing appropriate regimes are chosen.

Most women can have HRT, though the following situations may preclude it:

- Current or recent breast cancer (although some severely affected women do have HRT under guidance from their oncologist and after a detailed risk–benefit multi-disciplinary team discussion)
- Current or recent endometrial cancer
- Undiagnosed vaginal bleeding (must be investigated first)
- Active or recent blood clot (deep vein thrombosis/ pulmonary embolism) or stroke, heart attack or angina; if you have had one a while ago or have a clotting disorder, you may be able to have trans- dermal HRT (patch, gel or spray) but this will need further thought and discussion
- Active liver disease (because hormones are metab- olised in the liver)

The following conditions may need careful discussion and assessment but shouldn't preclude any discussion of HRT:

- Strong family history of breast cancer or ovarian cancer
- History of blood clots
- Migraine with aura (transdermal HRT is usually safe)
- Uncontrolled high blood pressure (needs controlling first)
- Gallbladder disease (oestrogen may worsen, although transdermal HRT is usually fine)

Here's the bottom line: if you are struggling with perimenopause and think you may want to try HRT but are dismissed or declined treatment, please do your own research, and if needs be seek out another opinion. No, we should not be assuming that all women in their 40s and beyond can only experience symptoms and concerns linked to their hormones, and yes, the prescription of HRT must be practised safely – but there are far too many women being dismissed and given incorrect information right now.

Non-hormonal treatment options

For those of you who don't want, can't access or can't have HRT there are a handful of pharmacological alternatives. In Chapter 7, we will look at why HRT may support your ADHD brain – I can't promise any of the non-hormonal treatments will do the same, but we can at least empower you to know your options and try to reduce some of your perimenopausal symptoms at this challenging time.

Clonidine and gabapentin can be prescribed to reduce hot flushes, although they aren't without other possible side effects. Medications called SSRIs and SNRIs (commonly known as antidepressants) have also been shown to be effective at reducing vasomotor symptoms (hot sweats and flashes) in perimenopause.

Understandably, women can feel let down, misjudged or 'fobbed off' when a GP offers an antidepressant in menopause, but there is evidence that they are effective in reducing the physical vasomotor symptoms (hot flushes and sweats) of fluctuating oestrogen at this time. Specifically, medications can include paroxetine, fluoxetine and citalopram. A low dose of paroxetine (10mg) appears to have the strongest evidence at the time of writing. There are newer non-hormonal medications on the horizon (such as fezolinetant) but these are not in wide use yet.

Vaginal oestrogen products are locally acting and often considered safe even when systemic HRT is not. Vaginal oestrogen, which acts locally in the vagina and vulval tissue, is unlikely to give you enough additional oestrogen to ease the symptoms of your ADHD caused by fluctuating systemic hormones. I mention it here, however, because I see so many women suffering with urogenital symptoms who have been misinformed about their ability to use this treatment, which can be used with or without other systemic HRT therapies.

Lifestyle changes to support your perimenopause and menopause

There are also proven benefits of certain lifestyle measures for easing perimenopausal and menopausal symptoms. Reducing your alcohol and caffeine intake is essential, as both can exacerbate symptoms. As a perimenopausal woman myself I can say with confidence that if you haven't noticed this already, I'm pretty sure you will soon. Smoking has also been linked to earlier menopause (1–2 years earlier than non-smokers on average) and a more severe symptom profile (studies show higher rates of hot flushes, night sweats and sleep issues in women who smoke). Smoking also speeds up bone loss as we age and potentially reduces the efficacy of HRT.

While not part of British Menopause Society (BMS) treatment guidelines, research from a study by King's College London suggests that eating 30 different plant-based foods per week, especially fibre-rich foods, can significantly boost your gut microbiome.

The gut microbiome is the community of trillions of bacteria, fungi and other microbes living in your gut. These microbes aren't just passengers; we now know they actively influence digestion, immunity, metabolism, mood (much of the hormone serotonin is made in the gut), and even hormone regulation. Scientists now believe that a diverse and balanced microbiome supports overall health, while disruption (dysbiosis) can contribute to inflammation, hormonal imbalance, mood changes and metabolic issues. In turn, supporting a healthy microbiome can improve your estrobolome: the collection of gut bacteria that metabolise and regulate oestrogen.

Here's how it works:

➢ Oestrogen metabolism is broken down by the liver and excreted into the bile, eventually reaching the gut.
➢ Certain gut bacteria in the estrobolome can reactivate some of that oestrogen, sending it back into circulation; the rest is excreted.
➢ A diverse, healthy estrobolome may ensure oestrogen levels stay more stable. If your gut microbiome is disrupted, oestrogen recycling can become inefficient (too much/too little/erratic), potentially contributing to hot flushes, mood swings, bloating, or irregular cycles during perimenopause.

You can support your estrobolome by:

- Eating fibre-rich foods (vegetables, legumes, whole grains) to feed beneficial bacteria.
- Including fermented foods (yoghurt, kefir, sauerkraut) or probiotics in your diet.
- Limiting antibiotic overuse, highly processed foods and excess alcohol, which can harm your microbial population.

While most evidence for the link between a better gut microbiome and fewer menopausal symptoms is mostly associational rather than proven, it certainly makes sense to try and improve our dietary intake. My usual advice would be to ensure you are eating a varied, nutrient-dense diet and aiming for the following (preferably from your diet, with supplements if necessary):

- Calcium: 1,000–1,200mg per day, found in dairy, tofu, leafy greens, almonds
- Vitamin D: a minimum of 400iu or 10mcg per day, found in sunlight, oily fish, fortified foods
- Magnesium: found in wholegrains, nuts, seeds, leafy greens
- Protein: 1–1.2g per kg body weight per day, for muscle strength
- Omega 3 fatty acids: found in oily fish, chia, flax, walnuts
- Fibre: 25–30g per day, found in wholegrains, beans, lentils, fruit, veg, nuts, seeds
- B vitamins – B6, B12, folate: found in poultry, fish, eggs, dairy, leafy greens

Along with looking after your estrobolome and eating well, getting enough of these nutrients – particularly calcium, vitamin D and magnesium – is important for supporting your health, along with regular movement and, if possible, a degree of strength training. In addition, stay well hydrated and avoid as many ultra-processed foods as you can; your mind and body will thank you for it.

Hormonal shifts and how they impact the brain (including differences in the ADHD brain)

To fully appreciate how female hormones can impact the ADHD brain, it is important to understand that there are several known differences between the brains of ADHD and neurotypical individuals, both in terms of appearance and function, and new information is emerging all the time.

On learning this, the next question patients often ask is, 'why can't I have a brain scan or genetic blood test to diagnose my ADHD?' Brain and genetic differences in ADHD are very real but not specific or reliable enough yet to use brain scans or genetic tests as diagnostic tools. Comparing the test results of neurotypical people to those of people with known ADHD has helped scientists to identify themes, patterns and key differences, but there is no single sign yet that can reliably say yes, this person has ADHD. Presently, ADHD remains a clinical diagnosis based on globally accepted criteria – but who knows what the future holds?

The following sets out what is known so far about the ADHD brain (these findings describe average patterns seen across groups and do not apply to every individual with ADHD). Also bear in mind that more studies are needed and some are ongoing.

i. **Structural Differences (how it looks)**
   - Smaller total brain volume: On average, some studies show that children and adults with ADHD tend to have a slightly smaller overall brain volume, particularly in areas linked to

attention and impulse control. This is not universal and can be subtle.

- Delayed cortical maturation: The prefrontal cortex (responsible for executive function, impulse control and attention) tends to develop more slowly in individuals with ADHD, typically lagging by about 2–3 years.
- Differences in specific brain regions:
  - Prefrontal cortex (the management centre of the brain): Often differences in connectivity and function, leading to difficulties in impulse control and working memory.
  - Basal ganglia (including the striatum): Differences in connectivity, affecting motor control and reward processing.
  - Cerebellum: Differences which may contribute to difficulties in coordination, timing and attention regulation.

2. **Functional Differences (how it works)**
   - Weaker connectivity in attention networks: Reduced connectivity between the prefrontal cortex and other regions involved in attention regulation, such as the parietal lobe.
   - Overactivity in the default mode network (DMN): The DMN, which is responsible for mind-wandering and daydreaming, is less effectively supressed during tasks requiring sustained focus leading to distractibility.
   - Altered dopamine signalling: Individuals with ADHD often have altered dopamine signalling and receptor activity in areas related to motivation and reward (e.g. the striatum and prefrontal cortex).

3. **Neurochemical Differences (chemical messengers)**
   - Dopamine and norepinephrine dysregulation: These neurotransmitters (chemical messengers), which are crucial for focus, motivation and impulse control, function differently in ADHD brains.
   - Lower dopamine transporters or receptors in key areas: This may explain why stimulant medications, which increase dopamine and norepinephrine availability, are effective in treating ADHD symptoms.

4. **Differences in Brain Activity Patterns**
   - Lower activity in executive function areas: The prefrontal cortex shows reduced activation during tasks requiring sustained attention, working memory and self-control.
   - Higher theta-to-beta ratio in some EEG studies: Individuals with ADHD have shown increased theta (slow-wave) activity and reduced beta (fast-wave) activity in some studies, which may be linked to difficulties with attention and alertness.

How your hormones affect your brain

If you are born female (assigned female at birth), regardless of neurodiversity, oestrogen and progesterone interact closely with the chemical messengers in your brain. This is a well-studied neurobiological and neuroscientific process. It is not new, but it is wildly under recognised, discussed and often under served in standard clinical practice. Fluctuations and the ultimate decline in your oestrogen and progesterone levels during perimenopause and menopause mean that this neurobiological process is altered during this stage of life.

Dopamine

Dopamine is a chemical messenger that plays a key role in your brain's reward, motivation and executive function abilities (attention, focus, working memory, decision making, etc.) as well as emotional regulation. Other chemical messengers also have a role to play – norepinephrine, serotonin, GABA, glutamate, histamine – but for now, we shall focus on dopamine. Your brain has an estimated 86 billion neurons (nerve cells). Each of these can form thousands of connections, creating a network of over 100 trillion connections that are constantly signalling and reading messages and allowing us to function. For messages to 'jump' from one nerve cell to the next, a series of chemical messengers are required that are constantly being used and replaced by your brain and 'received' at sites known as receptors.

People with ADHD often have altered dopamine transporter function (DAT1) in the brain, meaning dopamine is cleared out quickly, reducing its ability to act and keep all these functions on track. You may also have dopamine receptors (D1, D2, D3) that are less sensitive or available, so even when dopamine is present it doesn't work as effectively on these receptors. The overall effect of these differences in your brain is less efficient dopamine signalling, particularly for sustained attention, motivation and executive brain function.

If you have ADHD, you are often unconsciously chasing dopamine activation to stimulate your brain. Not only does this help you feel good, but it also helps drive your brain's executive function. You may have difficulty focusing unless it is on something likely to activate dopamine pathways such as a new idea, hobby or a task that is deemed rewarding, interesting or urgent. Do you find you perform at your best under stress, just before a deadline? If so, you may well have spent a large part of your life in fight or flight mode because you are chasing dopamine just to function. Fight or flight mode is a state of hyperarousal of our nervous system that prepares the body to either confront (fight) or flee (flight) a perceived threat. Persistently chasing dopamine to instigate brain reward, interest or focus can push the body into this constant state of hyperarousal.

In some cases, this may have led you to chase dopamine from alcohol, caffeine, sugar, nicotine, drugs, gambling, crime or even confrontational relationships. You may take on too many tasks and overcommit because you crave the dopamine buzz of something new. This is not due to an innate badness, laziness or lack of willpower – it is a dopamine regulation issue, and frustratingly it's so often under recognised. This is why non-harmful dopamine rewards such as exercise can be your best friend when you have ADHD.

A key factor driving your changing ADHD and unmasking in midlife is the interplay between dopamine in the brain and fluctuating oestrogen levels. As you learn about this interplay, you may also now be able to recognise these effects at other points in your life when oestrogen has fluctuated, such as just before your period each month, after giving birth and in puberty.

Oestrogen

Oestrogen boosts your dopamine production and activity in the prefrontal cortex (think of this as the management centre) of the brain. This area is responsible for executive function (planning, timing, etc.), attention and working memory. When oestrogen levels drop for whatever reason (even just before a woman's period) dopamine availability (and other chemical messengers) is reduced and ADHD symptoms are likely worsened. This may manifest as:

- enhanced brain fog (already a symptom of perimenopause)

- forgetfulness in day-to-day tasks
- greater challenge in starting and completing tasks
- increased emotional dysregulation

Oestrogen can increase norepinephrine availability and the ability for receptors to detect it. Fluctuations in oestrogen can therefore reduce norepinephrine function and affect:

- arousal
- alertness
- mental stamina
- stress tolerance
- the ability to sustain attention

Oestrogen impacts the production and transport of serotonin in the brain, leading to:

- emotional dysregulation
- irritability
- impulsivity
- anxiety

Serotonin is the brain chemical we often elevate with anti-depressants (often SSRIs) so although I would never want you to be misdiagnosed as having anxiety and depression, the-oretically these medications can be somewhat helpful to some aspects of ADHD.

Oestrogen can also enhance glutamate signalling and acetylcholine activity, both of which support working memory, cognition (thinking) and learning. These functions of your brain are already at risk in ADHD due to dopamine deficits, and perimenopause consequently compounds this.

Progesterone

Progesterone also plays a part in exacerbating ADHD traits through its effects on chemical messengers in your brain.

Progesterone decline typically starts some years ahead of oestrogen decline in perimenopause. Progesterone breakdown products act powerfully on GABA-A receptors in your brain, the same ones activated by sedating medication and substances such as diazepam, sleeping tablets and alcohol. Activation of these GABA-A receptors have a calming effect, increasing feelings of relaxation and emotional stability. Progesterone loss indirectly also affects serotonin, dopamine and noradrenaline.

As progesterone declines in perimenopause this may lead to increased anxiety, interrupted sleep and irritability – all features of perimenopause but potentially heightened when you have ADHD. Many of these features of ADHD are somewhat expected by all women in perimenopause because, regardless of your neurodiversity, hormones impact all our brain messenger systems. In the next section, we will look at the well-known overlap between perimenopause and neurodivergent traits.

Common perimenopause symptoms that overlap with neurodivergence – and how to tell which is which

The overlap between perimenopause symptoms and neurodivergent traits can be so great that many women (and even clinicians) can start to get confused about what is really going on in midlife. This often means that yet again, you may be misdiagnosed as 'just' menopausal or with a mental health condition such as anxiety or depression, though of course women with ADHD and perimenopause can also develop depression and anxiety.

Commonly shared features between perimenopause and neurodivergence include brain fog, poor concentration, forgetfulness, inattention, irritability, chronic tiredness, difficulty sleeping, sensory overload and complete emotional overwhelm. Both can lead to loss of self-confidence, low self-esteem and a complete inability to tolerate anything new, particularly if it is deemed stressful.

I hear from lots of you who are concerned you may be unmasking neurodivergence at this already challenging life stage. Sadly, so many of you are met with doubt, criticism and dismissal not just from loved ones, friends and colleagues but also from clinicians. In Chapter 8 we will explore how you can navigate the doubt and dismissal you may face and arm yourself with the tools to push forwards.

Summary: how to decipher the difference or coexistence between perimenopause and ADHD

1. **Timing and history**
   - ADHD symptoms are lifelong, often noticeable in childhood or adolescence – may become more noticeable in perimenopause as mask slips.
   - Perimenopause symptoms typically start in the 40s (sometimes earlier) and fluctuate with hormonal cycles.

2. **Response to hormonal changes**
   - Hormone support (HRT) may relieve several perimenopause-related cognitive, emotional and physical symptoms.
   - ADHD symptoms usually persist regardless of hormone levels, although can improve with HRT once in perimenopause (See Chapter 7). Often requires reframing and change in behavioural strategies.

3. **Impact on functioning**
   - ADHD affects organisation, planning, time management and task completion across the lifespan.

- Perimenopause tends to highlight memory and cognitive issues that may worsen as menopause ensues.

4. **Lifelong challenges**
   - ADHD women may, on reflection, have always had struggles and felt challenged even if they worked excessively hard to get by.
   - The midlife struggles that come with perimenopause can compound the challenges that ADHD women may have always faced.

It is true that menopause, ADHD and anxiety and depression can share similarities in what midlife women may experience. Brain fog, poor concentration and memory, mood changes and fatigue are just the headlines of what you may be experiencing right now. While a diagnosis of depression and anxiety may be completely appropriate at times, it can also come at the cost of missing the underlying issue of ADHD. All middle-aged women will go through the menopause, yes, but not all menopausal women will experience it negatively; neither will we all become depressed and anxious. Nevertheless, this gender bias and somewhat unfortunate overlap in how women present at this life stage can delay the recognition of ADHD, because both patients and clinicians might attribute all changes to menopause, with or without a concurrent mental health disorder.

In short, a good, detailed history should provide more clarity. ADHD difficulties will have been lifelong even if subtle, masked or overlooked for years. Most of you will be able to say that you have always felt different or that you have felt exhausted just getting by in life. You may be able to look back at your childhood, teenage years and early adulthood and recount countless examples of how probable ADHD has affected the course your life has taken, including careers, relationships and opportunities, yet never felt able to raise this until now. It is key that you think long and hard about this when considering whether you may have ADHD.

In Chapter 5, we will discuss how to share this with your GP so you can help them separate the overlap, or acknowledge they can coexist, without falling into the trap of being dismissed or misdiagnosed. It is important that we spread the word that both ADHD and menopause can and do often coexist and make each other so much worse. This unfounded dismissal of women must stop. You are on this journey not only to seek validation and support for yourself but to empower all women to stand up for years of misdiagnosis and gender bias. Our daughters deserve it. You deserve it.

TL;DR – Chapter 2: From ADHD Life to Perimenopause and Menopause: What's Going on in My Body and Mind?

- **Neurodivergent women, especially with ADHD,** can be successful but often mask symptoms, leading to burnout.
- **Masking** involves perfectionism, multitasking and hiding struggles.
- **Strengths**: High empathy, creativity, intuition, problem-solving skills.
- **Challenges**: Executive function differences (planning), emotional dysregulation, low self-esteem.
- **ADHD in girls** often goes undiagnosed due to internalised symptoms.

  Many women get diagnosed later in life, often triggered by their child's diagnosis.

- **Burnout** is caused by chronic stress, imposter syndrome and hormonal changes (like perimenopause).

- **Parenting while neurodivergent** is tough, especially with executive function and sensory overload challenges.
- **Perimenopause** causes hormonal fluctuations that worsen ADHD symptoms such as brain fog, irritability and sleep issues.
- **HRT is the first-line treatment** for menopause (if safe), though many women face inconsistent care.
- **Hormonal shifts** impact brain chemicals, worsening ADHD symptoms.
- **Call to Action**: ADHD in midlife is often misunderstood. Better diagnosis, support and awareness are essential.

Chapter 3
When the Mask Slips – The Emotionally Dysregulated Burden of ADHD

Topics covered in this chapter:

- Why perimenopause/menopause can unmask ADHD
- The patient that changed how I see women and ADHD forever
- Living with increased emotional sensitivity, anger and overwhelm – including why history expects it of women
- How does emotional dysregulation challenge us all?
- The potential devastating effects of emotional dys-regulation in perimenopause/menopause
- Toolkit for making positive change and soothing habits to implement

In this chapter we will take a deeper dive into why perimeno-pause and menopause can be a pivotal point in your ADHD journey. We will specifically look at why the falling hormones and other challenges at this key life stage may unmask your ADHD and potentially lead to increased emotional sensitiv-ity, anger, overwhelm and difference in your executive func-tioning. I also want to tell you about a patient that opened my eyes on women and ADHD as a GP. Finally, I will provide you with a toolkit of tips for making positive change and some soothing habits you can implement to help you on your journey to a place of inner peace.

Why perimenopause/menopause can unmask ADHD in midlife

Let's start by recapping the role of oestrogen and dopamine on your brain in ADHD. I've repeated this several times throughout the book because it is a key piece of information, upon which most other things sit.

Oestrogen plays a key role in the production and effective use of the chemical messengers in your female brain. This is especially true of dopamine, which as you now know is critical in attention, motivation, emotional regulation and executive function (planning, memory and focus) of your day-to-day life with ADHD.

In ADHD, it is primarily the disruption to **dopamine** in your brain that causes a significant number of the associated challenges. As explained in Chapter 2, however, there are other chemical messengers that can also play a part when disrupted in perimenopause.

During perimenopause, your oestrogen levels fluctuate unpredictably, and in menopause, oestrogen drops significantly and remains low. Suddenly your brain is struggling to manage dopamine regulation even more than before thanks to these persisting fluctuations in oestrogen levels and their knock-on effects on dopamine production and use.

Prior to perimenopause and menopause, you have no doubt spent years masking your ADHD struggles by relying on routine and structure, overworking to stay organised, living on high alert with high social awareness, and constant analysis of your interactions before and after they've occurred.

You have likely thrived in the first half of your menstrual cycle when you have had more oestrogen and likely felt slightly less capable in the second half of your cycle where progesterone takes over – a part of your cycle known as the luteal phase. You are more likely to have experienced premenstrual dysphoric disorder (PMDD) or premenstrual syndrome (PMS) than your neurotypical peers due to your brain's sensitivity to hormonal fluctuation, and the impact of that fluctuation on your ADHD.

You may have also come to the realisation that you seem more sensitive to hormonal dips than many other women; this can become notable over time during your menstrual cycle, post-pregnancy or through your contraceptive choices.

You are probably only now, in midlife, realising the depth of the effects of hormonal changes on your overall wellbeing and brain function. If this is your lightbulb moment, take comfort in the knowledge you are not alone, and you were never crazy.

The patient that changed how I see women and ADHD forever

ADHD is a neurodevelopmental disorder, and it's hard for many people to understand that it hasn't 'just happened' in midlife. It is quite unsettling for loved ones and even your GP to realise it's been missed (in part by them) for so long.

I remember very vividly a patient I had seen numerous times over the course of many years as her GP, from childhood to adulthood. She had struggled with poor attainment at school and latterly had recurrent challenges with anxiety and emotional outbursts, resulting in difficulty holding down jobs and relationships. She had been on and off antidepressants and in and out of therapy but always struggled to maintain engagement with either strategy. She had at times self-medicated with drink and drugs and at others become very isolated. She frequently told me she was 'no good at anything' and 'a failure'. I so desperately wanted to help her feel better about herself, but I too was at a loss. It wasn't that I didn't look for answers – I was just inexperienced and ill-equipped to see what I was missing.

Fast-forward to the patient's mid-20s following a pregnancy; while undertaking her postnatal check she was extremely agitated and tearful, which is not uncommon in the postpartum period. What was unusual was her description of complete overwhelm at things she had previously managed. She reported new and severe differences in executive function: complete task paralysis, brain fog and an inability to plan or process, alongside worsening emotional outbursts and anxiety. She was screaming out for help, convinced she was an incapable and unfit mother. Until this point, I had spent every minute with her looking to successfully treat a mental health disorder or help her social circumstances – things I now realise were largely because of her undiagnosed ADHD. She had had treatment-resistant anxiety and depression for years and not once had we asked why.

Nowadays, treatment-resistant and recurrent depression and anxiety will always make me consider underlying ADHD and neurodivergence. In this particular 'oh my gosh' moment, I recognised that perhaps the postnatal hormone shift had caused this woman's mask to slip and screened her for ADHD. She's now formally diagnosed and medicated, and she cannot believe the difference this has made to her life. This distressed presentation could have happened as a result of postnatal depression, but considering her previous years of difficulties since childhood, it suddenly all made sense. She tells me she is forever grateful for that day the lightbulb came on and while I wish I had seen it sooner, I am thankful that those hormonal changes did in part unmask her ADHD so that we could get her the help and support she needed.

This patient is, alongside so many other women just like you, the reason I wrote this book. I want this book to change not just your ADHD perimenopause journey, but those of all the women like you and those yet to get here. As GPs and healthcare clinicians we are forever learning, but the truth is we don't just learn *for* you, our patients, we frequently learn *from* you. If I can ask one thing from you it's this: please chat with your GP and don't write them off. Share this book with others and let's ensure a move to more timely and compassionate recognition and care. I too have frustrations with the situation as it stands, but we can choose to be part of the solution, not the problem.

Living with increased emotional sensitivity, anger and overwhelm – including why history expects it of women

If you are a woman with ADHD, there are certain traits you will probably recognise, having battled with them on a recurrent basis:

- Emotional sensitivity
- Anger
- Overwhelm
- Executive function differences (sometimes referred to as 'executive dysfunction', though this term is falling out of favour)

All the above are extremely common, especially in women with ADHD, but are significantly compounded by the falling and fluctuating nature of oestrogen in perimenopause. You may or may not have managed to mask these traits previously but in times of stress or hormonal change that mask can be harder to hold onto. Of course, gender bias, society and many different cultural norms already expect women to be emotional, irrational and hysterical. This can mean all too often women are dismissed as being 'overly emotional', 'needy' or more likely to receive a mental health diagnosis.

Sadly, we don't need to look too hard in the history books to see how we got here. The word hysteria comes from the Greek 'hysteria' (ὑστέρα) meaning *uterus* (or womb). Ancient physicians believed women's physical and emotional symptoms were caused by a 'wandering womb' thought to drift around the body, pressing on organs and causing illness, fainting, or 'irrational behaviour'. From the Middle Ages to the Victorian era, 'Hysteria' became a catch-all diagnosis for women with symptoms that medicine couldn't explain: anxiety, seizures, depression, fainting, pain. This reinforced the belief that women were biologically unstable. Freud later linked hysteria to repressed trauma and subconscious conflicts, but still largely related it to women. Throughout the nineteenth century and into the next, women who expressed strong emotion or physical symptoms without clear cause were labelled 'hysterical' rather than being investigated properly. Some of you may feel this is still the case today, and in certain situations I cannot disagree.

Hysteria was finally removed as a medical diagnosis in the 1980 DSM (Diagnostic and Statistical Manual of Mental Disorders) but we are still seeing its aftermath in women's healthcare. Women remain more likely to have their symptoms dismissed, their pain minimised, and their symptoms attributed to psychological distress before physical causes are fully investigated. Studies show time and time again that women are less likely to receive adequate pain relief in emergency departments compared to similar presentations in men. If I have left you in any doubt, just think: when was the last time you heard a man described as hysterical? The concept of hysteria has reinforced a cultural association between being female and being emotionally unstable. This makes it harder for women to be taken seriously in healthcare, leadership, and even in personal relationships across almost all settings. In my opinion, most women have a hard time getting societal and medical support but those who are emotionally dysregulated are likely to be particularly disadvantaged.

So, what is really going on with emotional dysregulation and ADHD?

People often think of ADHD as a concentration issue, likely because of the name 'Attention Deficit Hyperactive Disorder' itself. That aside, it's important we recognise that for many people, especially women, emotional symptoms can be just as if not more prominent. There are tangible, neurobiological reasons for this. As a woman or younger girl, emotional dysregulation (overwhelm, tearfulness, irritability) may be the first thing you remember being flagged to your GP or school by loved ones (often parents). I suspect ADHD was not on the radar. Instead of these traits being recognised as ADHD-related, you may have spent years being told you are 'moody', 'dramatic', 'stressed', 'hormonal', or ultimately diagnosed with anxiety and/or depression. As a female with ADHD, you are less likely to show classic hyperactivity. Instead, you may have been frequently described as scatty, easily overwhelmed, or overly emotional. These are descriptions that quite frankly send shivers down my spine, because they are inaccurate representations and can lead to misdiagnosis of bipolar disorder or emotionally unstable personality disorder among others.

While you may well have one of these diagnoses alongside ADHD, many of you will be mislabelled and mismanaged for years, believing and having others believe that you are 'unfixable'. As we have already identified, you may have already recognised how changing hormones impact on your ADHD traits, particularly your emotional regulation. Too often, this is dismissed as 'being hormonal', and no one looks at the underlying neuroscience of hormones in the brain. This in turn minimises the underlying role of ADHD in emotional dysregulation. When you arrive at perimenopause in midlife, often unaware you have ADHD and certainly unaware of the neurobiological reasons why you can't control your emotions as you would like to, you are flung into further chaos by hormonal disruption of the other chemical messengers in the brain that impact our mood, such as serotonin, GABA and norepinephrine. ADHD in perimenopause is consequently a bit like a traffic jam of chemical messengers in the brain all going AWOL and trying to meet the needs of your 100 trillion plus connections and 86 billion neurons (see Chapter 2 for further detail). When we put it like that, it's a wonder any of us ever have a good day!

Overwhelm and ADHD

Overwhelm is one of the most common and distressing symptoms women with ADHD describe in midlife. Hormonal fluctuations in perimenopause add to this significantly. You may have just about managed to keep on top of things throughout your life, then hormone fluctuations unmask your ADHD and everything 'unravels'. This is overwhelm. It can feel like you are drowning without a lifeline. This is not a failure or a flaw, but a neurobiological event caused by an overloaded nervous system. When this happens, your working memory will become limited, time blindness will get worse and your ability to manage time will decrease. Completing tasks can feel impossible and small demands can feel like a huge ask.

Like an overloaded computer system with too many tabs open, your brain is freezing and shutting down. You may experience 'not feeling real' or not feeling fully present, avoidance of people or activities, or panic which can show up as rage and emotional outbursts of frustration.

How does it feel to be emotionally dysregulated with ADHD?

As a woman with ADHD, you may frequently become overwhelmed with emotions that feel big, fast and hard to control. You may well recognise some of the below:

- ➤ **Rapid emotional shifts**: going from calm to tearful, angry, or anxious in seconds.
- ➤ **Intense emotions**: feeling emotions more strongly than others, e.g. joy is exhilarating, sadness feels physically painful.
- ➤ **Difficulty 'turning down' feelings**: once triggered, emotions can take a long time to settle in a way that is hard for others to understand.
- ➤ **Rejection sensitivity**: a sense of being devastated by criticism, perceived rejection, or even neutral feedback, even if provided with evidence to the contrary.
- ➤ **Justice sensitivity**: a heightened emotional reaction to perceived or real unfairness that triggers the nervous system intensely.

Internally, these emotions may cause you to ruminate, overthink and overanalyse situations. This in turn will likely affect your self-esteem and even cause you to withdraw. Over the years you may acquire layers of shame and guilt, perhaps accompanied by flashbacks to outbursts you really wish you'd been able to avoid. Outwardly this may show up as you snapping, reacting, seeming visibly frustrated and, at times, in complete meltdown. The latter is difficult to manage within relationships, education or jobs.

How does emotional dysregulation challenge us all?

Living with someone who frequently experiences emotional dysregulation, whatever the cause, can be extremely challenging for all concerned. I start by noting this because I don't believe we can truly validate the neurobiological roots of emotional dysregulation in the ADHD brain if we use ADHD as an excuse for poor behaviour towards others. It isn't, and never should be, an excuse. I know many of you will regularly feel mortified by your emotional dysregulation, to the extent that you may even be withdrawing from social settings, romantic relationships and friendships, and your self-esteem may be hitting rock bottom. I've seen it time and time again. I want you to know that there are neurobiological and tangible reasons why emotions are harder to regulate with ADHD. This is not to excuse it but to hopefully provide an understanding to support those affected and assist those nearby to handle it more productively. This next section covers the science behind emotional dysregulation; as you read through it, try to imagine the magnification applied when all this preexisting emotional dysregulation meets the hormonal flux of perimenopause already described.

The ADHD brain and emotional regulation

Warning: here comes the science!

ADHD involves differences in the prefrontal cortex (which regulates impulses, perspective and emotions), the amygdala and the limbic system in the brain (where emotions are generated such as fear, anger, frustration). In ADHD the prefrontal cortex is often underactive and matures more slowly, the amygdala is hyperactive, and other areas that regulate conflict and emotions show altered connectivity. Dopamine and norepinephrine (important chemical messengers in the brain) both become dysregulated in ADHD, meaning emotions are felt strongly, but the 'brakes' to regulate them don't always kick in effectively. A part of the brain called the DMN (Default Mode Network) is often overly active in ADHD, leading to an overplaying of events, heightened emotional memory and difficulty avoiding emotional triggers. The cumulative effect is your body activating 'fight-or-flight mode' and overreaction. Serotonin and GABA chemical messengers play a smaller role, normally helping you to feel calmer, but in ADHD brains their functional ability is reduced, meaning it's much easier to become irritable, angry and slow to calm down.

Your ADHD brain may also struggle with the ability to self-soothe, put things into perspective and control impulses. As I mentioned in Chapter 2, this may mean you live more of your life in a state of fight or flight, while needing extra dopamine activation to function and achieve (see page Chapter 1). Existing in this heightened state may help you finish your to-do list, but it also means your emotions can feel overwhelming and may spill out quickly.

Brain science aside, our environment and experiences play a huge part in how we react and respond to any given situation as we move through life. You may have spent years being misunderstood, criticised, or having to overcompensate. If this describes your experience, you likely have resultant increased emotional sensitivity and a heightened ability to detect perceived threat from others. This might show up as a sixth sense that alerts you to when someone is being disingenuous or poses a threat to you in some way, which can be used positively in so many situations. In Chapter 1, we noted how some research suggests neurodivergence may have been evolutionary and this intuition is a huge part of why that may be the case. In our current age, when we are not hunting for food or being hunted, it can perhaps be more difficult to manage. Emotional dysregulation is not an 'add-on' to ADHD, but is closely linked to the relationship difficulties, burnout, low self-esteem, and higher rates of anxiety and depression often seen in women with ADHD. This is especially true when the mask slips in perimenopause, and you can no longer hold it all together as you once did.

The effects of emotional dysregulation in perimenopause and menopause

Emotional dysregulation during perimenopause and menopause does not mean, as some clinicians and people say, just being in a bad mood, and ignoring it can have real consequences. In 2023, the overall female suicide rate in England and Wales reached the highest level since 1994 (5.7/1,00,000). The highest rates are among women aged 45–54 years, with some studies citing one in six perimenopausal women having experienced suicidal thoughts. While we have no specific data for suicide rates in women who are perimenopausal and have ADHD, we do know that adults with ADHD are already five times more likely to attempt suicide compared to those without. The lived reality that pushes women towards suicidal ideation is clear to see:

- Feeling like your brain has stopped working (and losing hope it will ever get better)
- Sudden loss of coping strategies that once worked
- Overwhelm and exhaustion, both physically and emotionally
- Increasing and intensified emotional dysregulation and burnout
- Feeling dismissed and not believed
- Loss of relationships, roles and support networks as things 'unravel'

This data proves that not only should we be recognising and validating the lived experience of ADHD, but we should also be offering tailored support for it. Towards the end of this chapter, I will provide you with some techniques to self-soothe and support your emotional overdrive.

How differences in your executive function of your brain feed into emotional dysregulation

We talked about your brain's effects on your executive functioning in Chapter 1; as a recap, think of the executive function part of your brain like the head office of a large organisation, sitting in the prefrontal cortex part of your brain. The office staff manage planning, time awareness, memory and tasks. The HR department of the head office is your emotional regulation, managing your impulse control and emotions and ultimately how you respond and behave. In ADHD, the head office staff take more breaks than they are entitled to, and when they are tired and overwhelmed, they often go on strike. The result is that you can do things properly when everyone is pulling their weight, but it isn't consistent and things like stress, overwhelm and tiredness (going on strike) exacerbate the situation.

We have talked at length about how oestrogen enhances dopamine and norepinephrine production and signalling in the prefrontal cortex (the brain's head office). We know that during perimenopause, oestrogen levels fluctuate and gradually decline, which reduces this chemical messenger support. ADHD is already characterised by lower dopamine and norepinephrine activity in these brain regions; the hormonal changes create a 'double whammy'. Head office tasks become harder to execute as a result, HR go AWOL and emotions spill over.

It isn't all about oestrogen, though; the breakdown

products from progesterone (allopregnanolone) enhance GABA (another chemical messenger), which influences calmness and emotional regulation. During perimenopause, progesterone swings can destabilise mood and increase irritability, stress reactivity, and overwhelm. Perimenopausal sleep disturbance adds to the chaos, and when tiredness kicks in, executive function is often the first thing to break, whoever you are. As hormonal support in your brain dwindles, those compensatory strategies demand more effort and often start to fail. As things get harder to overcome and your mask slips, the palpable mismatch between what you could once manage and what feels impossible right now lowers your self-esteem and increases your sense of failure. In turn your emotional regulation may be harder to keep in check. Have you ever tried to start, focus on or complete a task under emotional distress? It's no wonder the head office of your brain is in meltdown.

Your toolkit for making positive change

8 ways to soothe overwhelm

1. **Understanding and validation**
   Practise recognising when you feel overwhelmed. Using phrases such as *'This isn't me being dramatic, it's my ADHD brain processing emotions differently'* reduces shame.

   Sharing this with partners, colleagues or friends can also help them understand your reactions are about intensity, not intent.

2. **In the moment strategies (when emotions surge; takes practice)**

   ➤ Externalise the emotion: e.g. 'I'm angry / I'm

overwhelmed'. This activates the prefrontal cortex, creating a tiny bit of distance and time to process.

➤ Ground yourself: learn some breathwork or relaxation techniques. I like the five-sense check-in: 'What can I see, hear, smell, taste, touch?' to reconnect with the present moment.

➤ Static movement such as stretching can clear excess adrenaline.

➤ Body-based resets: cold water on the wrists, lying flat on the floor, rocking, weighted blanket.

➤ Predictable anchors: same calming music when working, same mug for morning tea.

➤ Using a 'buffer' before replying to emails/ messages or in arguments: e.g. 'I'll get back to you in an hour', 'I just need time out'.

3. **Daily regulation habits (let routine build resilience)**

➤ **Exercise:** helps regulate dopamine and stress hormones, especially rhythmic movement (walking, cycling, dancing).

➤ **Sleep:** stabilises mood swings and improves executive function.

➤ **Mind–body practices:** build in some self-compassion time to focus on you with practices such as yoga, tai chi, or short, guided meditations.

➤ **Sensory regulation:** weighted blankets, music, hot showers – set time aside to provide soothing inputs for the nervous system.

4. **Psychological therapies (depends on local provision and personal finances)**

➤ **CBT (cognitive behavioural therapy):** Helps reframe spirals of shame or rejection sensitivity.

> ➤ **DBT (dialectical behaviour therapy)**: Originally for borderline personality disorder but very effective for ADHD emotional dysregulation. Can teach you distress tolerance, emotion regulation and interpersonal skills.

> ➤ **ADHD coaching**: Practical, future-focused support for managing triggers in work/home life. Try to find someone that comes recommended.

5. **Medication (relies on a formal diagnosis and access to a prescriber)**

> ➤ Stimulant-based ADHD medication (methylphenidate, lisdexamfetamine) can reduce emotional volatility by strengthening the prefrontal 'brakes'.

> ➤ Non-stimulant ADHD medication (atomoxetine, guanfacine, clonidine) sometimes helps more with the emotional side than focus.

Neither medication is curative for emotional dysregulation but in some people they can help 'turn it down' a notch so other strategies are easier to use.

6. **Hormonal considerations**
   If you suspect that hormones are impacting how you feel, tracking your period against the intensity of your emotions can highlight patterns that can potentially be managed or at least anticipated. Adjusting ADHD or hormonal medication (if relevant) around these shifts can sometimes help. Having said this, we need more research in this area and a lot of what we attempt may be trial and error. See Chapter 6 to learn more about what we do and don't know about medications for ADHD in perimenopause.

7. **Connection and compassion**

   ➤ Have at least one safe person who 'gets it' and is protective.
   ➤ Build on your self-compassion. You can't expect others to understand if you don't model it yourself.

8. **Nervous system soothing**

   Overwhelm is often a dysregulated nervous system asking for relief. To soothe it you need to shift from fight or flight back to calm and safety. Here are some ways you can do this:

   - Splashing cold water on your face.
   - Practise breathwork: inhale for four counts then exhale for six. This helps stimulate the calming vagus nerve and reverse fight or flight mode.
   - Ground through the senses: five things you can see, four you can touch, three you can hear, two you can smell, one you can taste.
   - Humming can also lightly stimulate the vagus nerve.
   - Weighted pressure or self-holding can help: cross your arms and squeeze your shoulders or press your hands against your chest or thighs.
   - Nervous system micro doses: take 30- to 60-second pauses throughout the day – sip a warm drink and focus on the sensation, feel your feet on the ground, look out of a window.

General tips to help with executive function

ADHD brains are prone to overwhelm and then shutdown. Here are a few more techniques that can help keep executive function ticking over and steer you away from emotional meltdowns:

1. **Help your brain manage day-to-day life**
   - Use the 'Two-Minute Rule': if something that needs doing takes less than two minutes, do it now. For longer tasks, divide them into tiny steps that feel achievable e.g. instead of 'clean the kitchen' try 'clear one surface'.
   - Choose one focus for the week such as hydration, sleep, or tidying – not all three. Do everything in small steps.
   - Use trackers on keys, wallets, phones – don't expect your brain to remember where everything is or may have been left around the house.
   - Keep everything external, not just in your brain:
     - Use visual cues (sticky notes, whiteboards, fridge lists)
     - Start a brain dump journal; no structure needed, just unload
     - Try digital tools with alarms like Google Calendar and Notion, or structured to-do apps like Tiimo and Structured

2. **Look after your physical wellbeing**
   - Start the day with gentle, light movement: low-stimulation activity (not emails or social media) to gently awaken the brain function.
   - Boost dopamine in healthy ways: try something new like a new walking route, playlist, or pen. Play games, do puzzles and allow creativity without productivity pressure. Track small wins visibly with sticker charts, habit trackers, or checklists.
   - Look after your physical health: hydration, blood sugar balance, regular fresh air and movement. It is easy to get lost in your mind and forget these vitals.

3. **Be kind to yourself**
   - Compassionate self-talk: shaming yourself serves no purpose and shuts down motivation. Self-kindness builds resilience. Accept you are facing challenges that anyone in your position would find hard. Let go of perfection and celebrate your effort, not necessarily the outcome.
   - Connection through body-doubling and peer support: it's often tempting to isolate yourself, but growth will come from learning to live again your way, not shutting yourself away.

4. **Simplify**
   Do whatever you can to simplify your day-to-day. There are several tips throughout this book to suggest how. The key is to reduce the mental load and create clarity. Tell yourself that good enough is good enough. Move away from perfection; it likely serves you no purpose at this stage. Give yourself permission to change how you do things to suit your brain. You no longer need to live this way, constantly swimming against the tide.
   - Use the 'rule of one': do one thing at a time. Multitasking is not a productive operation in ADHD. It usually serves only to make everything unproductive.
   - Choose your three daily priorities and make everything else optional.

5. **Time and task management**
   This is a particularly hard ask for your ADHD brain. Getting this under control, or at least better control, can be a game-changer.
   - Use practical help such as timers. Try the Pomodoro technique; a time-management

method where you work in focused bursts followed by a timed short break (25 mins work/5 mins break) and repeat.
- Body-doubling: Have a friend, partner, or online group present while you do a task.
- Consider doing hard tasks during your high-oestrogen window (early in the cycle) when possible.

Make a love bag

Whether it's self-love or to give someone else, the following can be a little package of calm to carry:

- Noise-cancelling headphones or earplugs
- Soft blanket or weighted lap pad
- Lavender or peppermint oil
- Fidget toys or textured objects
- Journal or doodle pad
- Breath cards or visual grounding prompts
- Positive affirmation

By now I hope you can see that the name 'attention deficit hyperactivity disorder' doesn't come close to covering the issues faced by those with ADHD, and even less so for those who are experiencing ADHD in perimenopause. There are so many layers to the complexity of this situation that there is no one simple fix, but my hope is that bit by bit this book can arm you with the knowledge, insight and self-discovery to navigate the challenges that you are facing. In the next chapter we will focus more specifically on the hormonal changes in perimenopause and menopause and how these can start to affect other aspects of your daily life such as cognition, sleep, sensory experiences, mood and attention. Long-term coping strategies often fail under these hormonal changes, leading to ADHD symptoms becoming more visible ('unmasking'). We will also delve a little deeper into why recognition is such an important part of your journey, even if you choose to self-manage your ADHD.

TL;DR – Chapter 3: When the Mask Slips – The Emotionally Dysregulated Burden of ADHD

1. **Midlife Challenges and Diagnosis Difficulties**
   - Midlife brings added stress: work demands, caring for family, sleep problems and hormonal symptoms compound difficulties.
   - ADHD symptoms overlap with menopause symptoms (brain fog, mood swings), causing misdiagnosis or delayed ADHD recognition.
   - Many women only realise they have ADHD during midlife due to hormones, other stressors and a period of self-reflection.

2. **Emotional Dysregulation and Societal Bias**
   - Emotional sensitivity, anger, overwhelm and executive function differences are common ADHD traits worsened by hormonal changes.
   - Historical gender bias (e.g. 'hysteria') leads to women's emotional symptoms often being dismissed or misdiagnosed.
   - ADHD brain differences affect emotional regulation centres, causing rapid and intense emotions, rejection sensitivity and difficulty calming down.

3. **Impact on Life and Executive Function**
   - Emotional dysregulation can harm relationships, lower self-esteem and lead to withdrawal or burnout.

- Executive function (your brain's 'head office') struggles due to hormonal changes reducing dopamine and norepinephrine support.
- Falling hormones plus stress and sleep issues compound to result in worsening focus, planning, and emotional control.
- This gap between past abilities and current struggles lowers confidence and increases emotional overwhelm.

Chapter 4
How Hormonal Changes in Perimenopause Can Worsen Your ADHD Challenges

Topics covered in this chapter:

- How hormonal change exacerbates cognitive and sensory symptoms
- Sleep, mood, attention and overwhelm
- Toolkit: daily habits, lifestyle tips

So far, we've explored how you may have masked with ADHD throughout your life and how perimenopause and midlife challenges may have led to you unmasking. In this chapter, I will explain why being perimenopausal with underlying ADHD poses a cumulative challenge to your general cognition, sensory symptoms, attention, mood and sleep. Finally, this chapter will provide you with a toolkit for daily habits and lifestyle tips that may help when you have ADHD in perimenopause.

How hormonal change exacerbates cognitive and sensory symptoms

As we covered in Chapter 2, it is not groundbreaking or new science that the brains of those born female are affected by hormones. We have known for decades that hormones such as oestrogen, progesterone and testosterone have a significant role to play in our brain's executive function and even neuroplasticity (the brain's ability to change and adapt). So why does it feel like a revelation to so many of my colleagues? Why do basic biology classes in mainstream education barely scratch the surface of hormones beyond their use in reproduction? Why do we not routinely acknowledge this when we see women in healthcare, including in mental health? It is basic neuroscience, yet we are routinely leaving women and clinicians unprepared to join the dots. Let me do this for you right now.

During perimenopause, levels of oestrogen and progesterone fluctuate and eventually drop. These hormones (especially oestrogen) have a strong interactive and enhancing effect on brain chemical messengers such as dopamine, norepinephrine and serotonin which directly impacts on your sensory loading and your cognition (brain function). Hormonal changes during this time can significantly worsen cognitive and sensory symptoms in underlying ADHD. This seems to be especially the case if you have masked your symptoms (knowingly or unknowingly) up to the point of your hormones going haywire.

Cognition refers to the brain's processing of information to help you think, learn, remember, problem-solve and focus. During perimenopause, falling hormone support for the brain means cognition can be more of a challenge, creating problems such as brain fog, memory issues, difficulty making decisions or managing previously easy to navigate tasks.

Oestrogen not only has a positive effect on the production of chemical messengers like dopamine and serotonin, but it is also known to be neuroprotective. This includes supporting brain cell survival, stimulating growth of new connections (especially in the part of the brain which forms memories) and enhancing blood flow and therefore energy supply to the brain. When oestrogen levels drop, you may suddenly find things you previously did with ease and without thought become fatiguing and overwhelming.

In ADHD, this fatigue and overwhelm can be significantly more noticeable. Oestrogen boosts dopamine (among other chemical messengers) within the prefrontal cortex of the brain. As we've seen, this area of the brain is responsible for focus, memory and task mobilisation. When your oestrogen levels drop, the result can be reduced dopamine and a consequent decrease in memory and ability to task switch and follow the flow of conversation or written work. Unsurprisingly, considering everything we now know, this is even more noticeable with ADHD than with perimenopause alone.

Chemical messengers boosted by oestrogen (and likely to drop in peri/menopause)

Oestrogen doesn't act like a chemical messenger itself, but it strongly influences how several key brain chemical messengers function:

1. **Serotonin**
   - Oestrogen increases serotonin production.
     - ➤ Upregulates serotonin receptors.
     - ➤ Slows serotonin breakdown.
     - ➤ Supports mood stability, emotional regulation and sleep.

2. **Norepinephrine (noradrenaline)**
   - Oestrogen enhances availability and receptor sensitivity.
     - ➤ Improves alertness, focus and energy.

3. **Acetylcholine**
   - Oestrogen boosts acetylcholine synthesis and receptor activity.
     - ➤ Supports learning, memory and attention.

4. **Glutamate**
   - Oestrogen enhances glutamate signalling (but too much may also contribute to sensory overload when levels fluctuate).
     - ➤ Strengthens neuroplasticity, cognition and learning.

5. **GABA (gamma-aminobutyric acid)**
     - ➤ Oestrogen modulates GABAergic pathways (the brain's main calming system).
     - ➤ Helps with anxiety regulation, sensory sensitivity, emotional regulation and sleep.

Other brain benefits of oestrogen:

- Neuroprotection – supports cell survival.
- Myelin support – helps maintain nerve insulation for faster messaging.
- Neurogenesis and plasticity – stimulate growth of new connections, especially in the hippocampus (memory hub).
- Blood flow and glucose metabolism – improve brain energy supply.

Sensory gating and overload

As briefly discussed in Chapter 1, if you have ADHD or suspect you have ADHD, you may notice you often experience sensory processing sensitivity. This can manifest in several ways including becoming irritable with noise (particularly indiscriminate background noise) or discomfort with certain textures including those in food or fabric. You may also notice you get easily overwhelmed in busy environments such as supermarkets or shopping centres or feel sensitive to certain lights, smells or temperature changes.

When perimenopause hits, the drop in oestrogen can affect something called your 'sensory gating' and worsen your sensory symptoms. Sensory gating helps you ignore noise and other stimuli that you don't need to be aware of. Think of it as a filtering process for your senses. Oestrogen dropping may affect the brain's ability to filter out unnecessary sensory input and makes the inputs that get through feel harsher and harder to tolerate. There are some other factors that come with perimenopause that make sensory overload more likely. Women in perimenopause often have poorer sleep and rapid mood shifts, both of which can lower sensory tolerance. The result can be unexplained irritability and overwhelm.

Below, I've listed the chemical messengers in your brain that are involved in sensory processing and how both perimenopause and ADHD can affect them. This is heavy on the science, so you can skip over it if you'd like to:

Dopamine

- Regulates how sensory stimuli are prioritised; enhances sensory signals that are rewarding.
- Oestrogen enhances dopamine synthesis, release and receptor sensitivity. During perimenopause, fluctuating or declining oestrogen can destabilise dopamine function.
- In ADHD, dysregulated dopamine signalling may cause reduced ability to filter sensory input. Sensory seeking or distractibility may intensify.

Norepinephrine

- Increases the brain's response to incoming sensory input. Heightens vigilance and attention to environmental changes.
- In perimenopause, oestrogen and progesterone

modulate norepinephrine activity; fluctuations can make norepinephrine signalling unstable.

- In ADHD, this instability can cause emotional reactivity and hyperarousal. You may become more sensitive to noise or touch. You may struggle to maintain focus on relevant stimuli when signalling is unstable.

GABA

- Filters and dampens sensory inputs to prevent overload. Helps the brain focus on relevant stimuli by downgrading less important ones. Keeps the senses in check.
- During perimenopause, progesterone levels fluctuate, reducing GABAergic calming effects or making them unstable.
- In ADHD, this can lead to reduced downgrading of unimportant stimuli, resulting in sensory overload or impulsive responses. It can also affect sleep, causing disruption and increased agitation and anxiety, which can worsen sensory difficulties.

Glutamate

- In simplistic terms, mediates sensory signals from sensory organs like the eyes, ears and skin to the brain. Also plays a key role in amplifying sensory input and forming sensory memories.
- In perimenopause, lower or fluctuating oestrogen can lead to glutamate over- or underactivity, particularly in the prefrontal cortex.
- In ADHD, this can contribute to increased cortical excitability and overstimulation, and poor filtering of sensory input. This effect contributes to the anxiety and irritability linked to sensory inputs.

Serotonin

- Stabilises sensory input and emotional responses to stimuli (senses coming in) and influences the thresholds for sensory inputs such as pain, touch and sound sensitivity.
- In perimenopause, oestrogen supports serotonin synthesis and receptor function. Fluctuations in oestrogen can cause instability in these thresholds.
- In ADHD, this contributes to heightened emotional sensitivity to sensory stimuli, irritability and low tolerance to sensory stressors like pain, noise and touch.

Acetylcholine

- Helps the brain focus on important sensory information and ignore irrelevant information.
- In perimenopause, reduced or fluctuating oestrogen impacts the efficiency of cholinergic neurons (those that rely on acetylcholine) and this may affect sensory filtering negatively.
- In ADHD, this may contribute to reduced sensory filtering and reduced attention and focus to relevant sensory inputs. This can increase distractibility.

Essentially, the combination of perimenopause and ADHD creates amplified sensory challenges. As a result, you may notice greater sensory overload (light, sound, touch) and more emotional reactivity to everyday stimuli.

Sleep, mood, attention and overwhelm

Sleep

Sleep is a complex biological process relying on sleep-wake homeostasis (the body's tracking of its need for sleep), circadian rhythm (your internal body clock) and several key hormones: melatonin, cortisol and GABA (the calming chemical messenger). Oestrogen and progesterone play an important role in sleep regulation by enhancing and supporting all these processes.

How oestrogen and progesterone impact sleep

Oestrogen boosts serotonin and GABA, which helps calm the brain and lead to sleep. It also helps regulate body temperature and supports your circadian rhythm (internal body clock). As oestrogen falls in perimenopause you may feel more anxious and on edge, you may have hot sweats and night sweats, and your sleep may be disrupted. As progesterone drops, its natural calming effect on GABA receptors may be lost, leaving you potentially feeling more restless, agitated and more sensitive to stress. Falling oestrogen can also adversely affect melatonin production. The resulting effect of less oestrogen and progesterone is less time spent in deep restorative sleep and more frequent awakenings.

ADHD and the sleep–wake cycle

You may also struggle with sleep for very tangible reasons to do with your ADHD. Contrary to popular belief, it is not quite as simple as just struggling to 'switch off'. We've already talked a lot about the altered brain chemistry in ADHD, imbalances or altered function in several of the chemical brain messengers including dopamine and norepinephrine. Dopamine, norepinephrine and GABA are key players, responsible for the sleep–wake cycle. Disruption can lead to the ADHD brain struggling to move easily from awake to asleep. These brain chemicals are responsible for alertness, arousal and the sleep–wake cycle and because of their imbalance, you may notice a tendency for your ADHD brain to be more alert at night with what we call a delayed sleep phase.

The Delayed Sleep Phase Syndrome (DSPS) and Delayed Sleep–Wake Phase Disorder (DSWPD)

Are you the night owl in your family? Delayed sleep phase syndrome (DSPS) – otherwise known as delayed sleep–wake phase disorder (DSWPD) – is another term I want to introduce you to. Essentially, this describes a state when the internal body clock runs late. If you have DSPS or DSWPD you will likely feel naturally sleepy very late (2–4am) and wake naturally late morning (10am–12pm). In ADHD, melatonin production is delayed later than 'the norm'. This is common in other forms of neurodivergence, as well as depression, and can occur naturally in teens and young adults. Many people with ADHD have a delayed circadian rhythm (internal body clock) and altered sleep patterns (REM patterns). If this is you, you likely feel most alert in the evening, even if you feel physically tired. You may experience restless sleep and difficulty transitioning between sleep stages (from deep to light sleep for example). Of course, you may still have to wake early in the morning to get on with life, and this can lead to chronic sleep deprivation. It is true that your ADHD brain may well also struggle to sleep due to hyperactivity, and in women this tends to manifest internally as a 'racing mind', especially at night when distractions are less. We know that most ADHD brains struggle to move between tasks and transitioning into sleep mode can be another example of this.

Other factors that can affect sleep in ADHD

While there are neurochemical reasons for poor sleep, there are also some behavioural ones. The impairment to your executive brain function in ADHD likely impacts your time management and consistent bedtime routines. A consistent bedtime routine allows for winding down; this period of relaxation is so important for anyone to get a good night's sleep. With ADHD, sleep hygiene is often poor at best and missing at worst – the toolkit at the end of this chapter is designed to help you improve this.

Sensory sensitivity in ADHD, as discussed in the 'sensory gating and overload' section of this chapter (see page 81), may also play a role in difficulty getting to sleep; sensitivity to light, noise and temperature can all keep you awake. You may also find yourself seeking a dopamine boost from stimulation when the rest of the world falls quiet, and for many this means the dreaded doomscrolling late into the night. For those of you already on medication for your ADHD, this can be a double-edged sword where sleep is concerned. Stimulant medication can delay sleep in some cases, especially if taken too late in the day – for others it can help reduce your hyperactivity and restlessness, therefore aiding sleep. Be mindful that medication could well be having an impact on your sleep in either direction; discuss this with your specialist if you are concerned.

Sleep deprivation is not good news for anyone's mental or physical health; in ADHD it can worsen inattention, sensory overload, emotional dysregulation, brain function and impulse control. In perimenopause it can exacerbate brain fog, poor working memory and mood instability. Together, these effects can be debilitating but in the toolkit on page 91 you can find strategies that will hopefully help.

Mood

Oestrogen has a positive boosting effect on serotonin and dopamine. These brain chemicals help regulate your mood. As oestrogen fluctuates so too do serotonin and dopamine levels, potentially leading to an increase in anxiety, irritability, low mood and rage. This amplifies the preexisting emotional dysregulation that already exists with ADHD and which we explored at length in Chapter 3.

Emotional dysregulation in your ADHD brain is caused by a complex mix of neurological, chemical and structural factors. You will know by now that ADHD is essentially a difference in the brain's executive function. In short, this is the brain's ability to self-manage and plan. This extends to its ability to emotionally self-regulate. Being able to emotionally self-regulate shows up as being able to pause before reacting, reframe distressing thoughts or assumptions and calm yourself when your internal distress is escalating. Struggling to do this is not an irrational personality trait or poor self-control, in simple terms, it is your ADHD brain having inefficient or inconsistently activated areas in its prefrontal cortex responsible for these capabilities

How time blindness and rejection sensitivity impact emotional reactivity

Someone once told me that those with ADHD had only two time zones: now, and not now. I have absolutely found this to ring true on so many occasions. The technical term for this is 'time blindness'. You may find that your brain spends most of its time in the 'now'. Your brain lacks the capability to plan or think outside of now, which means that a current emotion, conflict or issue can feel permanent and fatal. This, of course, intensifies these moments and makes it difficult to establish perspective. 'This too shall pass' is a common comforting phrase you may find difficult to take on board in your ADHD stressed brain. You can also return to phrases like 'This moment is hard, but I'm safe' or 'This feeling is loud but not permanent'.

Do you experience extreme emotional pain from perceived criticism or rejection, known as RSD (Rejection Sensitive Dysphoria, common in ADHD)? Things that others may laugh off or not think much about can cut you deeply to the core for days, weeks or months. As outlined across the first three chapters, it is a self-fulfilling phenomenon, because as you experience repeated negative feedback (perceived or otherwise) during school, work and relationships, your emotional triggers are likely to become cumulative and generate a more intense response. While friends and colleagues around you seem to mellow with age, you may do the opposite, leading to embarrassment and shame at your frequent tendency to 'lose it'. Emotional resilience with time may not come as intuitively to you as it does to others, despite having strong natural intuition. Your gaps in working memory may also make it harder to notice when you are becoming emotionally overloaded. You can read more about this in Chapter 3 (page 62).

The upshot of all of this is that emotional dysregulation in ADHD often leads to you having outbursts, meltdowns and shutdowns that affect your relationships, your decision-making ability and, in many cases, can lead to misdiagnosis of mood disorders. Throw on a sprinkle of perimenopausal mood instability and you are heading for surefire crisis without any intervention. I hope you and those around you can use this book as part of that intervention. With understanding comes acceptance, and with acceptance come solutions. At the end of this chapter, we will discuss some possible strategies to help manage emotional reactivity.

Attention

It is a misconception that everyone with ADHD has a bad attention span. In fact, I prefer to think of it as attention difference, not deficit. You may well be able to focus – even hyperfocus – on things you derive great interest and reward from but struggle to maintain focus on tasks that seem dull or repetitive and ultimately don't boost your dopamine-seeking brain.

Having said this, we know that many women and girls tend to show inattentive type ADHD traits rather than the classic hyperactive impulsive pattern outwardly seen in many (though not all) boys with ADHD. The bottom line is: attention is likely inconsistent in women with ADHD rather than absent, and can be greatly altered by emotions, hormones, sleep, stress and overwhelm.

You will know by now that oestrogen is neuroprotective, meaning it supports our brain function. Oestrogen supports dopamine and acetylcholine transmission (for memory) among other things, so declining oestrogen will result in reduced cognitive clarity. This is why symptoms of perimenopause and ADHD can appear similar or overlap, such as forgetfulness, brain fog, reduced focus, slower processing speed and difficulty starting and completing tasks (see Chapter 2 for more detail on this). You may also have noticed that your focus and cognitive function have declined somewhat in the run up to each menstrual period as your oestrogen levels dip, or maybe you are just starting to piece this together right now.

The Default Mode Network (DMN) and attention in ADHD

The DMN is a large-scale brain circuit that essentially acts as our background operating system, constantly running programmes in response to things such as losing focus, daydreaming, thinking to ourselves, making plans and thinking about what has gone before. In ADHD, the DMN tends to be overactive (or rather less suppressed when concentrating), which can lead to the mind wandering during tasks, difficulty keeping focus, distractibility, repetitive internal monologue and poor working memory. This has been demonstrated in the brain MRI scans of those with ADHD. In a neurotypical person, the switch from DMN to TPN (Task Positive Network) is more efficient and leads to a much smoother transition between thought processes and subsequent tasks. Oestrogen fluctuations in perimenopause may destabilise this process, meaning attention switching often worsens. If you are also juggling high cognitive load (things to do, places to be and remember and so on), as many women in midlife are, the DMN can become even more overactive and intrusive, making attention much worse. This lack of attention can add to your sense of overwhelm – you can read more about this in Chapter 3 (page 63).

This overlap between the changes in the brain during perimenopause and unmasking ADHD often leads to clinicians, loved ones and even women themselves assuming that their attention switching abilities worsening is all just part of 'the change'. The truth is that experiencing perimenopause and ADHD simultaneously has a cumulative and often very debilitating effect on a woman, as we have explored throughout this book so far. Fluctuating hormones in perimenopause can not only unmask existing deficits and difficulties, but they can also compound them.

This is not you 'losing it'. This is your ADHD brain traversing perimenopause.

Toolkit: managing your sleep, mood, attention and overwhelm

I have no overnight fix for the challenges you are facing but like any dutiful GP, I do have a toolkit of suggestions for daily habits and lifestyle changes you can adopt to ease the burden. Some of these may be more likely to support your sleep, some of them your mood and some, like exercise, may help more than one of these things. If you are super keen to get cracking right now, you may be fighting the urge to hyperfocus on this list and try to implement every single one, before dawn. I recommend you take your time. Start low and go slow, building these into your life in a sustainable and enjoyable manner. You do not have to do them in any order, so start with those you feel most able to achieve first to build your confidence.

At the end of this toolkit, I share the generic 'sleep hygiene' advice that GPs and hospitals everywhere will reiterate. I don't expect you to feel able or willing to implement all this straight away – and some of it may never feel achievable – but I've included it here for you to think about. I know some patients feel like they are being fobbed off with generic sleep advice that seems too basic for what they are experiencing, but medicine has come so far in such a short time that we often skip over the simple things that can really make a difference. This book is here to offer you the whole scope of what may help you, from simple to aspirational. You are believed here, and I have no doubt you can make great improvements to your life. Progress is made the moment you take that first step.

1. **Maintain Consistent Wake-up and Sleep Times**
    - Aim to wake up and go to bed at the same time daily, even on weekends.
    - This will help to stabilise your circadian rhythm (internal body clock).
    - Consider using light alarms or sleep apps if mornings are a struggle.

2. **Use a Visual To-Do List**
    - Keep it visible (whiteboard, sticky notes, app with widgets).

- Prioritise just 1–3 tasks per day. Any more than this is likely overwhelming.
- Break big tasks into micro-steps so each task becomes a series of small actions you can achieve. E.g. instead of 'write report', say 'open laptop and title report'.

3. **Time-Block Your Day**
   - Schedule tasks into chunks of time (e.g. 9–9:30: email, 9:30–10: meeting).
   - Blocking out time helps to combat time blindness and improves transitioning between tasks.
   - Use digital calendars, alarms, or even physical timers to prompt you when it's time to move on.

4. **Schedule Regular Eating**
   - This may sound simple but hyperfocus and time blindness commonly lead to lack of food. Time may run away from you and suddenly you feel starving.
   - All brains, but especially those with ADHD, need steady glucose and protein to function efficiently.
   - Irregular eating worsens blood sugar control which causes significant fluctuations in mood, irritability and focus.
   - Keep easy nutritious snacks available (e.g. nuts, protein bars, fruit) at home or work.

5. **Move Your Body Daily**
   - 10–20 minutes of intentional movement boosts dopamine and therefore executive brain function.
   - Walking, dancing, stretching – anything that gets you moving will help.
   - Even 1–2 minutes of movement between tasks can reset your brain. This is a concept known as

exercise snacking; doing little bits throughout the day that all add up. It is a concept backed by research, shown to improve your health and wellbeing in several ways including your brain and memory health.

6. **Use the 'Body-Doubling' Technique**
   - Work alongside someone else (in person or virtually) so they keep you on task. The body double does not need to actively participate in the task; their presence alone provides accountability and a sense of structure and framing.
   - This is great for starting tasks you are resisting and staying on track with support.

7. **Join an ADHD Community and Engage**
   - Being able to express yourself with others in similar situations, facing similar challenges, can be unbelievably therapeutic. Don't knock it until you've tried it.

8. **Have a Morning and Evening Routine**
   - Keep routines simple and repeatable (in the same order each day). An example may look like:
     - Morning: wake, drink water, take meds, eat, plan day.
     - Evening: shut down work, prep for tomorrow, wind down (screens off, lights low).
   Sticking to routine helps the ADHD brain to reduce overload, emotional overwhelm and decision fatigue. Your brain takes a lot of effort to plan, initiate, organise and remember next steps. Repeatable routines (even for other things like what to have for dinner each day) can help reduce

the pressure on it. It may seem harder at first, but it will get easier as the routines become familiar.

9. **Pre-Decide Your Day**
- ADHD brains burn energy on making decisions. Reduce decision fatigue by:
  - Setting out clothes
  - Prepping meals or snacks
  - Blocking the day in advance
  - Whatever else you can do to be ready for the incoming day

Of course, these things can be a challenge whenever they are undertaken which is why number 8 in this toolkit – keeping routines – can assist with this.

10. **Add One Minute of Mindfulness**
- Not a long meditation – just a pause, whenever you feel one is needed. Do this at frequent intervals throughout your day.
- Before switching tasks or when overwhelmed, stop and:
  - Breathe.
  - Notice your surroundings.
  - Ask: What's the next small thing I can do?
  - Remind yourself you are not failing, broken or incapable.

11. **Limit 'Digital Drift' (otherwise known as doomscrolling)**
- Use screen limiters, app blockers, or visual cues to reduce social media rabbit holes and YouTube spirals.
- Try 'phone-free first hour' or screen curfews at night. Setting an alarm to signal the end of scrolling time can help.

- Lots of ADHD resources discuss this and what to use and how.

12. **Reward Yourself Often**

Motivation can be interest-based in ADHD; use small rewards after completing tasks to keep your dopamine-seeking behaviour on track. Your ADHD brain will look for dopamine hits where it can, so ensure you choose healthy options that you control to avoid getting sucked into others like excess alcohol and gambling.

13. **Declutter Your Space**

Keep your space decluttered to avoid taking up brain space with 'visual noise' and becoming overstimulated and overwhelmed. Every unnecessary object in your room, on your work desk, and in your handbag competes for your attention. It requires constant filtering of irrelevant stimuli which zaps your focus. Get rid.

Sleep hygiene advice

Sleep hygiene is not specific to ADHD but it's something we should all be doing to assist a good night's sleep. These things can be harder to implement with consistency if you have ADHD, but I'd encourage you to do what you can. The section on sleep earlier in this chapter explores the knock-on effects of poor sleep in perimenopausal ADHD; here are the NHS guidelines on how to practise good sleep hygiene.

1. **Create a restful bedroom environment**
   You can do this by:

- keeping the room temperature at a comfortable level (a very warm room is more likely to disrupt your sleep)
- keeping the room as dark as possible

- keeping the room as quiet as possible or using earplugs

2. **Only use your bedroom for sleep, sex and getting dressed**
   Avoid watching television, listening to the radio or reading in bed. This will help your brain to recognise your bed as a place for sleeping.

3. **Stop using electronic devices before going to bed**
   This includes computers, smartphones and televisions, as they can all stimulate your brain for several hours after use, making falling asleep difficult.

4. **Avoid stimulants after lunch**
   Caffeine can take up to six hours to wear off, so avoid anything containing caffeine after 2pm. This includes coffee, tea, energy drinks and chocolate. It may also include your stimulant medication if you forget to take it earlier. Nicotine is a stimulant and will keep you awake, so avoid smoking and vaping before going to bed. Alcohol may make you feel drowsy, but it does not improve sleep quality and will make you need the toilet more often than usual, which will disrupt your sleep. Avoid drinking alcohol before going to bed and try not to rely on it to help you fall asleep.

5. **Eat a light meal before going to bed; avoid heavy meals in the evening**
   Going to bed too full can force your digestive system to keep working when it should be resting. Likewise, going to bed hungry can also disturb your sleep.

6. **Exercise regularly during the day**
   Exercising during the day can help you have a better night's sleep. However, vigorous exercise within

three hours of going to bed may delay your sleep. Try doing a relaxing form of exercise before going to bed to help you sleep, such as yoga or stretching. Walking is also great for gentle regular exercise that can also get you outdoors and moving. It doesn't have to be far; a walk around the block after lunch or dinner is a great start. Building in little bits of extra movement like parking further away from the supermarket can soon add up.

7. **Get regular exposure to natural light**
   Morning and early afternoon light exposure will help you to maintain a healthy sleep-wake cycle. Too much light exposure in the evening can prevent you from feeling sleepy.

8. **Create a relaxing bedtime routine**
   When you are stressed or anxious, your body produces more cortisol (the stress hormone). Give yourself one to one and a half hours to wind down before going to sleep. Try meditating or having a warm bath before going to bed.

9. **Limit or avoid taking naps during the day**
   Staying awake during the day will make you more likely to fall asleep at night. Taking a nap late afternoon or in the evening is likely to affect the quality of your night-time sleep. If you do take a daytime nap, this should be no more than 30 minutes.

10. **Use technology to your advantage**
    Suggesting you look to technology for help may seem a little counterintuitive when much of this chapter asks you to get off your screens, but they do have their place and new apps are coming out all the time. See the Resources at the back of this book for suggestions.

By now, you should have a sense of exactly what's going on in your brain with ADHD and perimenopause and, perhaps more importantly, how this impacts your day-to-day functioning and emotional regulation. The next chapter will guide you in taking these concerns and insights to your GP to ask for help. I shall give you my insider's view as a GP of how best to approach it, what to say, what to expect and how to get past any stigma and disbelief you may face. Going to your GP to say you think you may have ADHD or perimenopause, not least both, can be anxiety provoking but together, we can work through how to tackle it head on, because you deserve to be validated and supported.

TL;DR – Chapter 4: How Hormonal Changes in Perimenopause Can Worsen Your ADHD Challenges

How Hormonal Change Exacerbates Cognitive and Sensory Symptoms

- Oestrogen and progesterone support brain function; their decline worsens ADHD symptoms.
- Perimenopause impacts memory, focus and decision-making, especially in women who've masked ADHD for years.

Sensory Gating and Overload

- Hormonal shifts reduce sensory filtering which leads to more overwhelm.
- ADHD and perimenopause increase sensitivity to light, noise and touch.
- Key brain chemicals (dopamine, GABA, serotonin, etc.) become dysregulated, heightening sensory overload.

Sleep, Mood, Attention and Overwhelm

- Hormone loss disrupts sleep, raises anxiety and worsens emotional regulation.
- ADHD brains often have delayed sleep cycles and difficulty winding down.
- Mood swings and rejection sensitivity increase; attention becomes harder to control.
- Common signs: feeling burnt out, forgetful, easily triggered, or 'not yourself.'

Toolkit: Daily Habits and Lifestyle Tips

- No instant fixes but can build slowly and sustainably.
- Improve sleep hygiene, manage sensory inputs, set routines.
- Avoid overwhelm; pick one habit at a time.
- Self-awareness is your first and best step to coping better.

Chapter 5
Talking to Your GP When You Think You Have ADHD

Topics covered in this chapter:

- Preparing for a productive conversation – six steps prior to your appointment
- What are your referral options (including Right to Choose providers, prescriptions and shared care agreements)
- What to do while you wait for assessment
- What to expect in an assessment or referral
- Navigating stigma, disbelief, or limited services

When you suspect (or in many cases know) you have ADHD, it can be hard to know what to do next, and specifically how to broach it with your GP. I am often asked by women how they can get their GP to take them seriously. Some of you may have already tried and been dismissed and some of you I suspect are anticipating being dismissed or, even worse, worried about being made to feel stupid. I can't promise you that your GP will listen or act, but there are things you can do beforehand to give yourself the best fighting chance. I know it shouldn't be this way (and it isn't always) but when you experience difficulties during those initial steps it can be soul destroying, so I want you to be prepared.

Preparing for a productive conversation

Here are six key steps I recommend undertaking prior to your appointment. You may be reading this having already got a diagnosis of ADHD but perhaps feeling like perimenopause has derailed you. As such, you may recognise some of the pitfalls we are about to explore, and in Chapters 2 and 7 you can learn about how to get help more specifically for your perimenopause too. For those of you approaching a GP about ADHD for the first time, some of this advice was covered briefly in Chapter 1 but here we will go into each step in detail to guide you in this important part of your journey.

1. **Do your research**

    The irony of asking you to do some research when you likely find it difficult to focus and complete tasks is not lost on me, but sadly the referral and assessment process can be challenging for those who likely have ADHD. It is not that you are not capable, but the difference in your brain's executive function means that you may feel complete overwhelm at the prospect of starting and completing a raft of paperwork.

    It's time to buckle in and channel your hyperfocus into learning about ADHD symptoms in adults, and especially women (inattention, emotional dysregulation, RSD, function differences, etc.). Weave into this knowledge about common coping mechanisms such as masking (see Chapter 1) and consider how these symptoms and coping strategies have affected or continue to affect your daily life including your work, school and relationships. The earlier chapters in this book should have hopefully helped you with this but you can also use reputable information from sources like ADHD UK. A list of resources can be found at the back of this book.

Be mindful that ADHD in adults is not widely known about in any great depth by many clinicians, including some GPs. You may well come across a clinician who wrongly believes you cannot be successful and have ADHD, that you cannot have ADHD as you were not disruptive at school or in trouble with the police, or that you cannot 'present' in adulthood. These are all real-life examples I have heard numerous times from women who have subsequently been dismissed. It is important you are armed with information to refute all these common myths calmly and factually. If this is something you may struggle with, I'd encourage you to involve a loved one who is willing to learn with you and attend your GP appointment to advocate for you. A clinician should be fine with someone supporting you in an appointment if you are happy for them to be there.

2. **Screen yourself for ADHD across your lifespan**
There is no single test that a clinician can do to diagnose ADHD. It is a clinical diagnosis based on comprehensive assessment by a specialist. This consists of a detailed history, a series of symptom checklists and questionnaires, relevant observations from others and clinical judgement. There are globally accepted diagnostic criteria that need to be met to finally settle on a diagnosis after this thorough assessment. Most UK clinicians use the DSM-5-TR criteria (as discussed in Chapter 1) which requires:

- Several symptoms to be present before age 12
- Symptoms present across two or more settings (school, work, home, etc.)
- Clear evidence of interference with day-to-day life (in relationships, work, education)

- Symptoms that cannot be better explained by another condition

Your GP or an ADHD specialist is likely to first perform a basic ADHD screening questionnaire, such as the Adult ADHD Self-Report Scale mentioned in the first chapter. It makes sense to do this yourself before you present to your GP asking for referral. Signposting to this is available on the Resources page.

Alongside this, try to write a journal of your struggles back to childhood; symptoms should have started before age 12 but often women have masked their entire lives and present in later adulthood, notably perimenopause (see Chapter 2), so this may need some thought and explanation. If you can, it may help to chat to parents, siblings, dig out old school reports. I always find it amazing what family members and loved ones come to accept as run-of-the-mill traits until questioned. Provide specific examples of how your symptoms impact your life. Even if you appear to have your life in order, it can be exhausting to get to that place while compensating. Many women have lost relationships, friendships, jobs or even their self-esteem along the way. Get ready to spell this out to your GP.

3. **Book an appointment with your preferred GP**
   I'm sure it is no secret that GPs vary massively in their approach, experience, interests and even their demeanour. If there is a GP you know and trust, or one with special interests in neurodivergence or menopause, at your practice then I'd always recommend waiting to see them. You are likely to have to wait and this may seem frustrating, but the chances are you have waited your whole life to get

to this point, so personally I would hold out for the GP you feel most comfortable with or who you feel may be the most helpful. If you can book a longer appointment (often called a 'double' appointment), even better.

I have a supportive interest in women with ADHD, so I will always listen and try to understand women's struggles. When my patients aren't aware of this, it's not uncommon for them to come in 'on the attack' for an assessment request. I understand why. You have probably spent a large part of your life feeling not enough or too much and you may well be tired and frustrated. You may have been fobbed off, dismissed, or misdiagnosed as you navigated life's stresses and challenges and now you are expecting to be badly treated, misdiagnosed, dismissed once again.

If I can offer one small piece of advice based on my experience, leave this baggage at the door. Go in open-minded, armed with information and practicality. When patients attend ready for a fight, for any reason, it's so hard to come back from and it rarely ends well for either party. Be prepared to discuss your life course and how things affect you: demanding a referral and expecting it without discussion won't help. It is a good idea to write things down if you are likely to get distracted or bring someone to support you who knows you well.

4. **Consider other factors**

It is true that many neurodivergent women are often misdiagnosed as having a mental health disorder throughout the course of their life. We have looked at why overlapping symptoms between perimenopause, mental health disorders and ADHD can make this more likely. Estimates vary, but studies suggest 20–50 per cent of adults with ADHD are initially misdiagnosed, often with depression or anxiety. Antidepressants can have inhibitory effects on some of the symptoms of perimenopause, such as hot flushes and unstable mood, but the first-line treatment in all guidance that clinicians are deemed safe to prescribe is HRT (see Chapter 2). I don't condone any woman being dismissed as solely anxious or depressed, but I do know that mental health disorders can co-exist with ADHD and do so frequently. In fact, living with undiagnosed ADHD often causes anxiety or depression due to chronic stress, underachievement, low self-esteem and strained relationships.

These secondary issues may be more visible and obvious when we aren't looking for the underlying ADHD. Many clinicians are more familiar with anxiety and depression than adult ADHD, especially in primary care. ADHD is also historically seen as a 'childhood disorder', so adult patients are not routinely screened for it. If you are a high-achieving woman, masking ADHD through overcompensation, perfectionism, or high effort, you are more likely to have hidden the core symptoms of ADHD. Be mindful of things coexisting and if you feel your clinician is attempting to push a diagnosis towards a mental health disorder, explore this with them too but be honest about your concern that the root cause here may be ADHD and why. Having ADHD does not exclude you from having anxiety and depression and vice versa.

5. **Directly ask for a referral**
GPs often use a communication tool called ICE; this stands for ideas, concerns and expectations. If

they feel it's relevant, they may try to elicit your ideas about what is going on, your concerns about it and what you expect to happen from this point onwards. Sometimes it may sound like your GP is asking you for the answers, but rest assured this is a tried and tested tool, to ensure we fully understand where you are coming from and ensure we don't leave you with unanswered thoughts or concerns. It works well providing you engage with the process and feel able to be open and honest with us. If you don't feel able, we may think we've addressed everything when we haven't.

To this end, I would recommend that you directly ask your GP for a referral for an ADHD assessment. Your GP does not have to refer you if they don't feel you may have ADHD but, in my experience, women have done a lot of research by the time they reach us, and we should not dismiss this. Be armed with the knowledge that ADHD can often go undiagnosed, particularly in adults or certain groups (e.g. women, non-hyperactive individuals). If your GP dismisses your concerns or won't refer you, ask them to explain why; remain calm but assertive. Politely emphasise the impact these symptoms have on your life and reiterate your request for an assessment. If your GP continues to dismiss you, you're entitled to seek a second opinion from another doctor. Of course, there is always the real possibility you don't have ADHD, but I expect if you are here and fully informed, this is somewhat unlikely.

6. **Know your referral options**
   Before you attend your GP appointment, try and have an idea of what referral options may be open to you for where you live. Most areas have an NHS

Adult ADHD clinic that GPs can refer into if they feel someone is suitable, but they often have long wait times. This also appears to be a postcode lottery, with some areas reporting waits of up to 10 years, and others having closed the waiting list due to complete overwhelm (how very ironic!). If you reside in England, you can consider asking for a 'Right to Choose' provider. This is an approved group of private providers, usually operating online, to which the NHS can refer you without passing on the cost to you. They often have shorter than local wait times (and the shortest can change from week to week, so it's worth keeping an eye on this). From time to time these lists will also close to allow the providers to catch up and further funding assessments from the health board. Information on the providers available, their wait times and scope can be found on the ADHD UK website (see Resources on page 209).

What are your referral options (including Right to Choose providers, prescriptions and shared care agreements)?

It is worth bearing in mind that many providers will want to hand any subsequent prescription for ADHD medications over to your GP and your GP may also not accept prescribing responsibility or shared care. I would urge you to have this discussion from the outset with your GP and ensure you understand the assessor's intentions before starting the process, if medication is something you are thinking about. Waiting years for an assessment, getting a diagnosis and then not being able to access treatment can be the last straw for some. Others may feel having a diagnosis is therapeutic enough.

What Right to Choose Covers (England Only)
If you're eligible (more on that below), you can be referred by your GP to an **RTC-eligible provider** for*:

- An **ADHD assessment**
- A **diagnosis**, if appropriate
- A **treatment plan**, which may include a **recommendation for medication**

What Right to Choose Does NOT Always Cover
Ongoing medication titration (increasing the dose over time and assessing effects) and prescribing are not always included in the RTC agreement; it depends on the provider.
Some RTC providers:

- Do provide full titration and handover to your GP once stable.
- Don't do titration and instead send a treatment plan to your GP, who is then expected to initiate medication and titrate it locally (which many GPs cannot do without specialist input or a shared care agreement, which they don't have to agree to – see below).

At the time of writing, there is a clear table on the ADHD UK website detailing what each provider offers and potential wait times.

Does my GP have to agree to a shared care agreement?

Shared care agreements are a way of specialists and the patient's GP sharing the care of specialised conditions that

* NB: at the time of writing some areas have temporarily paused RTC.

require specialised medication, for example ADHD, rheumatoid arthritis or inflammatory bowel disease (IBD). Usually, the drugs involved must be started and stabilised by a specialist.

The General Medical Council (GMC) and British Medical Association (BMA) are very clear that GPs are not obligated to take on shared care, and if a shared care agreement cannot be put in place after treatment has been initiated, the responsibility for continued prescribing sits with the specialist who started the medication. The specialist in turn may decide that they cannot provide the patient with prescriptions and monthly monitoring.

The reality is that this can leave you, the patient, stuck in the middle with no medication. While I understand this can be upsetting, it is usually due to safety reasons or concerns from the GP about lack of support or experience around the condition or treatment. Here are a few reasons why:

- GPs may feel they lack the specialist knowledge or training required to safely manage a particular medication or condition. If we prescribe it, we are responsible for it.
- Shared care treatments or conditions require ongoing specialist monitoring, which GPs may not be equipped to provide in a primary care setting. GPs may refuse shared care if they feel they cannot meet the standards of monitoring or treatment recommended by the specialist team, either because of knowledge, experience or capacity.
- Shared care protocols need to be clear, comprehensive, and mutually agreed upon. If the GP finds the arrangements unclear or inadequate, they may decline to participate due to the responsibility it involves. Equally, shared care protocols should allow the GP to obtain timely specialist advice and access

for the patient back into the specialist service. If this looks doubtful, the GP is less likely to agree to it.

- GPs are independent contractors and have the professional right to decide whether to accept specific responsibilities that aren't in the core contract, which includes shared care agreements. Every practice has different levels of staffing, resources, GP experience and confidence in local services so who agrees to what will vary.

Other options if a shared care agreement doesn't work out

As we mentioned above, if your GP does decline shared care, the responsibility typically remains with the specialist or hospital team that did the initial assessment and diagnosis, which ensures the patient continues to receive the necessary care. However, I have by now come across many cases where the original assessment clinic does not feel able to provide this service of monthly prescriptions and monitoring, which leaves diagnosed patients in limbo. If that happens to you, there are a few other options to look into.

Some areas may have a 'fast-track medication-only clinic' for those who have been assessed and diagnosed with ADHD (either privately or within the NHS) and need NHS prescriptions through their GP. While a new assessment to diagnose ADHD can take 2–3 hours, a medication initiation or titration appointment can be quicker and carried out by team members other than doctors, such as nurse prescribers and pharmacists. This means that there may be an NHS clinic separate to the ones diagnosing people that can see you, review your assessment and agree to start and titrate medication. In this scenario, some GPs may then feel more comfortable to continue prescribing and monitoring you from there, but again, they don't have to. You may find waiting lists for these NHS medication clinics are shorter, or you may find this set up doesn't exist at all in your area. Either way, if you do find yourself stuck, it's worth asking whether this option is available to you.

If there are no such services, or the answer is still no, then your options will be to pay privately for prescriptions via a private clinic, or look to manage your ADHD without medication, which hopefully the rest of this book can help with. I'm a firm believer that medication for ADHD *can* be an incredibly helpful stepping stone, a way of getting the brain better 'oiled'. However, medication alone is rarely the whole solution. Thriving with ADHD usually requires a wider framework of support around the person; a combination of supportive relationships, inclusive environments and tools that help regulate a sensitive nervous system.

What to do while you wait for assessment

The euphoria of finally being listened to and referred can be short-lived when you are met with lengthy uncertainty over when you will be formally assessed. If you are confident in the likelihood of an ADHD diagnosis, I would not let a lack of formal diagnosis deter you from seeking support and implementing tools that may help in the meantime.

Many of the ADHD support networks will be very welcoming to those who are still awaiting formal diagnosis or self-identifying as ADHD. Accessing support that may improve your day-to-day existence is harmless even if you turn out to not have ADHD. Support groups will largely focus on shared experiences, coping strategies and a sense of belonging and community. A full list of resources for support can be found on page 209.

Waiting for an ADHD assessment can feel like a mix of self-recognition, doubt, and even a surge of imposter syndrome about having ADHD. Many women report feeling anxious and worried, often more than they ever imagined. Going through an ADHD assessment can feel exposing and vulnerable. The possibility of a non-diagnosis result can stir up disappointment, self-doubt or even grief. This is not because you want to be labelled, it's because you want clarity on your years of torment. A clinician stating you don't meet all ADHD criteria does not erase your lived reality. Your experiences are still valid.

Here are three tips that may help you to feel steadier:

1. **Expect the doubts**

- Almost everyone going through this process has moments of 'maybe I don't have it' or 'maybe I'm exaggerating'.
- Those doubts are often part of the ADHD experience itself (second-guessing, overthinking, worrying about getting it wrong).
- Try to hold both possibilities lightly: you might meet criteria, you might not, but either way, you'll know you have done what you can to understand yourself.

2. **Prepare emotionally for both outcomes**

- If the answer is yes: you'll have a framework for understanding yourself and (if you want) exploring treatment or adjustments.
- If the answer is no: that doesn't mean you imagined your struggles. It may mean your challenges sit in the 'subthreshold' zone, or overlap more with something like anxiety, executive function differences, or autistic traits. You still deserve support.

3. **Remember the journey ends when you park up**

- If you don't get the outcome you are expecting, take

some time out to reflect and regenerate. Focus on self-care and compassion.

- Sometimes assessments miss things, especially if traits are masked, or they don't see the whole picture. You can seek a second opinion or revisit assessment later if difficulties persist.
- Focus on self-validation above any diagnostic stamp. Use the support tools if they help. A diagnosis may explain you, but it does not define you. Your struggles and your strengths are real either way.

What if I don't want to be assessed and formally diagnosed?

Some of you will remain 'self-identifying' – that is, you will continue to explore ADHD and be pretty sure this is you without a formal diagnosis. Many of you will choose not to seek a formal diagnosis at all. Some of you may already have a diagnosis and be here trying to bolster how you feel about things or find out what to do next. One of the most common groups of people who self-identify with ADHD is women who are in their adult years and navigating menopause. You can find more information on the pros and cons of getting a diagnosis as well as self-identifying in Chapter 6, coming up next.

Seeking an ADHD diagnosis as an adult can be costly, time consuming and emotionally draining, especially while also navigating hormonal imbalance. It is a very personal choice after a lifetime of reckoning.

I would encourage you to think about what a diagnosis would mean to you. Will it add validity and a sense of clarity to your struggles, or would you feel unnecessarily labelled? Do you have a workplace that may be able to support you better with a formal diagnosis or could you get along making changes yourself with support? Would you want to look at the possibility of medication? Or are you content learning about how the ADHD brain works and making the relevant accommodations? Everyone's circumstances are different and sometimes getting a formal diagnosis is not how you think it will be.

The option of seeking a private assessment

If NHS waiting times are long, you can choose to seek a private ADHD assessment. Costs for private assessments vary. There are a multitude of private ADHD assessors, and it can be overwhelming knowing who to choose. As an NHS GP, I'm expected to remain impartial and avoid endorsing one specific private provider over another. Please don't interpret this as me disliking or disagreeing with private care. You will most likely find that your GP is quite open to discussing private care as an option but will not recommend a specific service or specialist. My general advice is to ensure the private specialist is registered with the General Medical Council (GMC) or another regulatory body such as the Nursing and Midwifery Council (NMC) or the Health and Care Professions Council (HCPC) and clinics should be registered with the CQC (Care Quality Commission). Once again, be mindful that your GP may also not feel able to prescribe any medications you are given.

As already discussed earlier in this chapter, ADHD medications are specialist medications. They are mostly controlled drugs that need a shared care agreement for the GP to prescribe, which they are not always able or willing to do. In this case your only option is to pay privately for the medication, which is usually issued monthly. The cost of this will be calculated per tablet so, unlike on an NHS prescription, getting a bigger supply less frequently will not ease the financial burden. You will also need to engage in regular checks, such as your blood pressure and weight. This is incredibly important. As I mentioned further up, some areas offer NHS medication clinics that can manage prescriptions for those with a private ADHD diagnosis but be prepared to fund the monthly medication fee if being medicated is what you are aiming for. If you remain uncertain, you can navigate the pros and cons of seeking a diagnosis in Chapter 6.

What to expect in an assessment or referral

A formal ADHD assessment with a view to a new diagnosis can take up to 2–3 hours. This can be a challenge for your ADHD brain, but those undertaking such assessments will be fully aware that you are likely to encounter some inattention and hyperactivity challenges during the assessment. Most will start by putting you at ease, recognising the difficulties you may face with such a long assessment and offering you breaks when required. If this does not happen early on and may be an issue, I would raise this with the assessors as it is important you are as relaxed and focused as possible to get the most out of the assessment.

Prior to the assessment, you'll have been sent a series of questionnaires to complete. The assessment will involve a detailed discussion of your symptoms and medical history, as well as a review of the pre-assessment questionnaires and scales you have completed to assess your ADHD symptoms over your life course and settings. These pre-assessment questionnaires will usually also include information from others who know you well (e.g. family or friends).

It is important the ADHD specialist tries to rule out other conditions that could explain your symptoms. This can be triggering if you have spent large parts of your life feeling fobbed off or misdiagnosed by professionals. Hold your nerve, because this is not them trying to fob you off, this is them ensuring they have done due diligence. There are diagnostic criteria to be met. Usually by the end of the assessment, the clinician will be able to give you a good idea of what they think, and possibly a diagnosis.

Not everyone will be suitable for medication, or want medication, but this will also likely form part of the discussion along with other things that may help such as psychological support, ADHD coaching, or occupational therapy. Do not be alarmed if the specialist starts asking about your family history of sudden cardiac death among other things; this is a quick screen for your suitability for some of the common ADHD medications. Medication may not be your go-to; sometimes just having an answer and support is enough at this juncture.

What are the criteria to be met during assessment?

There are many reasons why women are often late to be diagnosed with ADHD, but one of them is the misunderstanding that an adult needs to be impulsive to have ADHD. In fact, girls and women are far more likely to have inattentive symptoms. According to DSM-5-TR (the diagnostic manual commonly used in many countries), ADHD can be diagnosed based on inattentive symptoms, hyperactive/impulsive symptoms, or both.

There are three presentations of ADHD (previously called 'subtypes'):

1. Predominantly Inattentive Presentation
2. Predominantly Hyperactive/Impulsive Presentation
3. Combined Presentation

Inattentive symptoms (need ≥6 for children, ≥5 for adults)

An individual often:

1. **Fails to pay close attention to details** or makes careless mistakes (e.g. overlooking or missing details at work).
2. **Has difficulty sustaining attention** (e.g. in conversations, reading, tasks).
3. **Does not seem to listen** when spoken to directly.
4. **Does not follow through on instructions** and fails to finish tasks (starts but gets sidetracked).
5. **Has difficulty organising tasks and activities** (e.g. poor time management, messy work).
6. **Avoids or dislikes tasks** requiring sustained mental effort (e.g. completing reports or paperwork).
7. **Loses things** necessary for tasks (e.g. keys, glasses, phone, documents).
8. **Easily distracted** by external stimuli (or unrelated thoughts).
9. **Forgetful in daily activities** (e.g. appointments, returning calls).

Hyperactive/impulsive symptoms (need ≥6 for children, ≥5 for adults)

An individual often:

1. **Fidgets with hands or feet**, taps, or squirms in seat.
2. **Leaves seat** when staying seated is expected (e.g. meetings, work).
3. **Runs about or climbs excessively** in inappropriate situations (in adults, may feel restless).
4. **Unable to play or engage in leisure activities quietly.**

5. **'On the go' or acts as if 'driven by a motor'** (e.g. can't relax, constantly busy).
6. **Talks excessively.**
7. **Blurts out answers** before questions have been completed.
8. **Has difficulty waiting their turn** (e.g. in queues, conversations).
9. **Interrupts or intrudes on others** (e.g. butts into conversations, may take over tasks).

Diagnosis requires:

- **≥5 symptoms** in either category (for adults ≥17 years old).
- Symptoms must be **present for at least six months.**
- Several symptoms must have been **present before age 12.**
- They must occur in **two or more settings** (e.g. work, home, social).
- They must **clearly interfere** with social, academic, or occupational functioning.
- Symptoms are **not better accounted for** by another disorder.
- **NB: Children** (16 and under) must meet six or more symptoms in either category.

For example, an adult that meets five or more symptoms from the inattentive symptom list may meet criteria for inattentive ADHD, and if they meet five or more from the hyperactive symptom list they may be diagnosed as hyperactive ADHD. If they meet five or more in both categories, they could have combined ADHD. The other factors listed above must also apply after a lengthy and detailed assessment.

Soft signs of ADHD are subtle indicators that may not meet full diagnostic criteria but can still suggest underlying attention or executive functioning challenges. These signs can vary by individual and may be mistaken for personality traits or other conditions in earlier years. Here are some possible soft signs:

Attention and focus

- Frequently zoning out or daydreaming, even during important conversations
- Difficulty following long or detailed instructions
- Often needing background noise or music to focus
- Struggling with reading long texts despite being interested in the topic
- Losing track of time easily, leading to lateness or rushed tasks

Memory and organisation

- Forgetting small but important details (e.g. names, appointments, due dates)
- Frequently misplacing everyday items (e.g. phone, keys, wallet)
- Needing reminders or alarms to stay on track with tasks
- Procrastinating even on things they want to do
- Difficulty prioritising tasks, leading to last-minute cramming or panic

Emotional regulation

- Feeling overwhelmed by frustration or impatience
- Being highly sensitive to rejection or criticism (rejection sensitive dysphoria/RSD)

- Frequent mood swings or difficulty regulating emotions
- Impulsive emotional reactions that are later regretted

Energy and restlessness

- Feeling constantly 'on the go' mentally, even if not physically hyperactive
- Having trouble relaxing or unwinding before bed
- Frequently tapping, fidgeting, or needing to move (even subtly)
- Periods of intense hyperfocus followed by complete exhaustion

Social and communication patterns

- Interrupting others unintentionally during conversations
- Difficulty remembering details from past conversations
- Struggling to maintain friendships due to inconsistent engagement
- Over-explaining or going off on tangents when telling a story

Many of these soft signs overlap with other conditions like anxiety, autism, or sleep disorders, so they aren't definitive for ADHD.

What if I don't get a diagnosis?

Being told you don't meet the criteria for a diagnosis of ADHD after a long, drawn-out wait can be heartbreaking. It's not that you want ADHD per se, but you know something is wrong and you want an answer. Acknowledge how you are feeling and know that it's ok and common to feel this way. It does not make you pathetic or needy, as I've heard other women claim. Remember the three tips I shared earlier in this chapter about how to frame things while anxiously waiting for an assessment; the essence of these can be extended to help you process this outcome.

My initial advice in this situation is to take a few days out to process the assessment. Sometimes what we hear in the moment and what was said are not the same thing. Sometimes women hear 'you do not have ADHD' when in fact the following may have been said:

- 'You don't meet the formal diagnostic threshold right now'
- 'Your difficulties might be better explained by something else (e.g. anxiety, trauma, autism, menopause, or other neurodivergence)'
- 'You show some traits but not enough for a diagnosis'

Ensure you receive a written summary of the assessment and clarity over which criteria you haven't met and why. I would also ask for the assessor's opinion on what else may be causing your difficulties if not ADHD, if they have not already offered this information. Saying you do not meet the ADHD criteria is not the same as invalidating your struggles or how challenging things remain for you.

It is important to remember that even without a formal diagnosis of ADHD, you may still self-identify as ADHD and many support resources and groups will remain open to you. You may feel the assessment didn't get a thorough picture of your challenges or needs, was rushed or unprofessional. You may want to ask for a second opinion – though let's face it, waiting for the first one was probably a marathon. Sometimes it can seem very likely that a woman has ADHD, but other overlapping conditions may be at play such as childhood trauma, autistic spectrum traits, menopause-related brain changes, and anxiety. A formal diagnosis does not define you, or how much support you require or are deserving of. Even without an ADHD diagnosis many women will still benefit from coping strategies, coaching or therapy, peer support and accommodations designed for those with ADHD.

Even if you're told you don't 'qualify' for a formal ADHD diagnosis, your lived experience still matters. Here are a few things that can help:

- Find community (online or in-person support groups)
- Use self-help tools for executive functioning and focus
- Work with a therapist or ADHD-informed coach who understands neurodivergence
- Journal or reflect on what strategies help you to manage daily life

Remember, you are always believed here.

I have a diagnosis: now what? Dealing with stigma, disbelief and limited services

Diagnosis is often a huge relief for women, but it is by no means the endpoint. Many women find what comes next to be just as overwhelming. If you have been recommended and assessed as suitable for medication, you may or may not be able to access this via the NHS. Ironically, despite the NHS not always providing the medication arm of treatment for ADHD, it is even less likely to provide ADHD coaching, therapy and access to occupational therapy. Navigating this constant battle with limited services, disbelief and stigma around ADHD can be emotionally draining and feel at times like you are stuck in reverse.

The reality is that ADHD services are underfunded and overstretched across most of the UK, especially for adults. ADHD is still considered a relatively 'new' area in adult psychiatry; many services were originally set up just for children. While perimenopause and menopause care has gained great media attention and traction over recent years, we remain a way off providing high quality and accessible menopause care for all women, let alone care and assessment for ADHD in perimenopause. My hope is that one day combined assessments and care are standard practice, but for now we must support each other and muddle through.

Part of that progress will hopefully mean eroding the stigma and disbelief that women face on a regular basis. Sadly, stigma is not confined to the public; some clinicians may also wrongly (in my opinion) dismiss ADHD as a 'current' or over-diagnosed condition. Chapter 6 discusses why I don't accept that ADHD and perimenopause is over-diagnosed or 'wanted' by women, and how you too can push back on this.

Here is a list of 'disbelief statements' I have been told by women with ADHD and how I would recommend responding to them:

- 'You're too successful/old to have ADHD.'
- 'But you went to university/have a job.'
  - Be sure to mention the hidden cost of this success: masking, burnout, anxiety, low self-esteem, sheer exhaustion.

- 'Everyone's a bit distracted these days.'
- 'That's just modern life.'
  - Acknowledge the above but also acknowledge the lifelong course of your issues and not just at times of stress or related to modern life.

- 'This is probably anxiety or trauma instead.'
- 'You don't need an ADHD label.'
  - Point out that coexisting conditions are common, and both can be true. ADHD often underlies lifelong anxiety. You are not looking for a label; you are looking for answers to your lifelong struggles.

- 'We don't have funding for this.'
- 'There's a long wait; we'll be in touch.'
  - Ask about Right to Choose (if in England), or request signposting to support in the meantime.

Receiving a diagnosis of ADHD can be debilitating initially. You may feel grief for lost time and opportunities, anger at dismissal and being misunderstood. You may feel frustrated with a service that is slow at best and limited at worst. The process of validation, healing and self-connection starts now.

You are not imagining it.

You are not broken.

You are not alone.

TL;DR – Chapter 5: Talking to Your GP When You Think You Have ADHD

Six quick steps

1. **Research ADHD**: Know the symptoms, myths and how it affects you. Bring someone to support if needed.
2. **Self-screen**: Try an ADHD questionnaire and note lifelong struggles with examples.
3. **Choose your GP**: Pick one you trust or who understands ADHD/menopause. Be calm and clear.

4. **Consider other issues**: ADHD often overlaps with anxiety, depression, or menopause symptoms. Be honest.
5. **Ask for referral**: Request an ADHD assessment directly. If refused, ask why and seek a second opinion if needed.
6. **Know your referral options**: NHS waiting lists can be long. In England, 'Right to Choose' private clinics may be faster but check medication support.

Waiting for Assessment

- Wait times are long.
- Use support groups and coping tools in the meantime.
- Be prepared for any outcome; your struggles are valid either way.

Don't Want a Diagnosis?

- You can self-identify and still benefit from understanding ADHD.
- Decide if a diagnosis will help or feel like a label that doesn't add much to your life.

Private ADHD Assessment

- NHS waits can be long; private assessments are an option but can be costly.
- Choose a registered specialist and clinic.
- GPs may not prescribe medication after private diagnosis; meds might need to be paid for privately on a monthly basis.
- The GMC and BMA support GPs if they don't feel able to agree to shared care agreements and prescribing.

What to Expect in ADHD Assessment

- Assessment takes 2–3 hours with questionnaires and interviews.
- Clinician rules out other causes and gives diagnosis based on multiple pieces of information.
- Discussion about medication and other supports (therapy, coaching) should be involved.

ADHD Diagnosis Basics

- ADHD presents in three types: inattentive, hyper-active/impulsive, or combined.
- Adults need 5+ symptoms in one category (inattention or hyperactivity) lasting 6+ months, starting before age 12, and causing problems in 2+ settings.

If You Don't Get Diagnosed

Not getting an ADHD diagnosis can be upsetting and that's understandable. You might hear things like:

- 'You don't meet the criteria right now.'
- 'Your difficulties may be due to something else.'
- 'You show some traits but not enough.'

Ask for a written summary and what else might explain your challenges. Your struggles are real even without a diagnosis. Support and coping strategies are still available.

Without diagnosis, you can still:

- Join support groups
- Use self-help tools
- See ADHD-aware therapists or coaches

After Diagnosis

Diagnosis is a relief but can feel overwhelming. NHS access to medication and therapy is limited, and stigma exists. People may say:

- 'You're too successful/old.'
- 'Everyone's distracted now.'
- 'It's just anxiety or trauma.'
- 'There's no funding.'

Explain masking, coexisting conditions and lifelong struggles. Ask about support options.

Remember: You're not imagining it, broken, or alone.

Now that you hopefully have a better understanding of what you are dealing with and how to approach it with your GP, what to expect in any given assessment and the aftermath, in the next chapter we will explore the pros and cons of seeking a diagnosis or choosing to self-identify. We will also look at the negative inner voice you may have acquired because of years of self-doubt and criticism, and how to change that and bring loved ones along with you (or not).

Chapter 6
Diagnosis or Self-Identifying Your ADHD in Perimenopause or Menopause

Topics covered in this chapter:

- The pros and cons of formal ADHD diagnosis in midlife (during perimenopause and menopause)
- Self-identification and self-accommodation
- Finding your own language (calling out your inner voice)
- Helping loved ones understand

Embarking on a diagnostic journey for ADHD at any age is not for the faint-hearted. In this chapter we will look at the pros and cons of an ADHD diagnosis for you. We'll explore the challenges of undertaking this journey alongside perimenopause, and how and why some of you may choose to go it alone and self-identify. I will then help you to find your own language in this space so that you can help your loved ones also develop a supportive understanding of you and your ADHD.

The pros and cons of formal ADHD diagnosis in midlife (during perimenopause and menopause)

If you are a woman seeking a diagnosis or recently diagnosed with ADHD, I can almost guarantee you will have been questioned by others, including clinicians, about why you would want a diagnosis at this point in life. In my experience, most of you have given the same response: because it will validate who you are and why you've struggled your whole life. Many of you will have reached this point due to the hormonal changes you're experiencing because of perimenopause, which are covered in detail in previous chapters.

While some of you seeking a diagnosis in midlife will be hoping to manage your ADHD with medication, I believe many more of you will just want an answer and to feel finally understood, not just by others but also by yourselves. Some of you will be unsure whether to seek a diagnosis or not and here, we will explore the pros and cons of doing so. The reality is that a formal diagnosis may open doors to ADHD support and services. Some of you may want to explore medication options to physically improve focus, energy and emotional regulation and you will most certainly require a formal diagnosis to do this. Medication comes with its own pros and cons, as discussed in Chapter 7.

Some of you may want to access NHS therapy tailored to ADHD such as CBT, coaching or support groups. Unfortunately, like NHS referrals for ADHD assessments, these too can be hard to come by. Those of you who have a formal diagnosis may feel better placed to access support in the workplace. While not all workplaces are aware of accommodations that can support neurodivergent employees, many do seem to be starting to look at and tackle this. A formal diagnosis may provide you with the confidence to open those discussions.

You don't need a formal diagnosis to learn about your probable ADHD but in my experience, it helps in the journey to self-discovery and inner peace. Not only does a formal diagnosis help you to seek acceptance from others, perhaps more importantly it helps you to seek acceptance from yourself. It may also help you understand why your perimenopause and menopause journey can feel different to others around you, or more specifically why you are 'unravelling'. There are also management and treatment to be considered when ADHD and perimenopause collide, and we will discuss these in Chapter 7.

On the topic of hormonal treatments, much research is still needed but we are starting to understand the nuances of how neurodivergent women may interact differently with and respond differently to hormones than we initially anticipate. It is important we identify neurodivergent women successfully and accurately, so we can continue to build on this understanding of hormonal therapy variances, and your healthcare team can manage women like you in the most supportive and effective way.

As a GP, I feel duty-bound to tell you that an ADHD diagnosis is not all positivity and awakening; so here come the downsides.

A late diagnosis of ADHD is still frequently met with societal stigma. It is not uncommon to hear rhetoric like 'everyone wants ADHD these days'. Wanting to be diagnosed to provide clarity and support for your lifelong suffering and wanting ADHD are not the same thing. Nevertheless, I still hear this ignorant remark far too often.

A diagnosis can be a huge relief, but it can also trigger complex emotions. I liken processing a midlife ADHD diagnosis to that of the Elisabeth Kübler-Ross stages of grief: denial, anger, bargaining, depression and acceptance. Just like the stages of grief, these emotions can arrive haphazardly, not always in a predetermined order or indeed when you expect them. A diagnosis can trigger any or all these emotions due to the sheer volume of opportunities, decisions and life paths that may have been different had ADHD been recognised for you sooner. It also comes from the recognition that many years have likely been spent overcompensating and consequently exhausted.

ADHD medication is not ideal for everyone. Even if your ADHD clinician thinks you are suitable and it may help, it can be a long journey to find the right medication and dose that suits you. Likewise, your GP may not agree and doesn't have to agree to prescribe your ADHD medications and if you chose to go down this road without them, it could prove costly. This can leave you feeling confused and abandoned. You can find advice on talking to your GP about an ADHD assessment, and why they may not prescribe ADHD medications for you, in Chapter 5, while Chapter 7 explores the topic of specific ADHD medication.

Being diagnosed in midlife is a personal decision and not one that should be taken lightly. I'd encourage you to enlist the support of someone you love and trust who can help support you throughout the process. The following lists outline the potential pros and cons of seeking an ADHD diagnosis in perimenopause/menopause:

Pros

- Clarity and self-understanding; making sense of lifelong struggles at a time when you feel hormonally stripped of your identity too.
- Becoming aware of ADHD and the effects hormonal change can have on ADHD may lead you to see your perimenopause, and how to manage it, through a different lens. I've met women who are more likely to turn to HRT due to the combined effect on their symptom profile of also living with neurodivergence.
- Access to ADHD specific medications, services and support (e.g. at work) and a better understanding of how your brain functions, especially with the coexistent impact of fluctuating hormones, can make you more proactive at seeking support.
- Integrating an ADHD diagnosis with your menopause care can help fine tune hormonal management based on how the neurodivergent brain may respond to hormones (albeit understanding of this is currently poor).

Cons

- Risk of over-attributing symptoms to ADHD when they may be purely hormone related, and vice versa.
- Perimenopause can muddy the water, making diagnosis difficult; women can feel invalidated if lifelong struggles are put down to current hormone changes or a definitive diagnosis is not provided.
- Some women don't tolerate new ADHD medications well while also perimenopausal, especially if sleep is already fragile. You may also have other age- or menopause-related risk factors that may mean meds are less suitable, e.g. CVD risks.
- May invoke a grief response about lost years and why ADHD wasn't picked up sooner.
- There is no standard clinical practice that assesses both ADHD and menopause or perimenopause as a dual concern and offers holistic assessment and management. This can make seeking diagnosis and validation a challenge and affect your self-esteem.

Of course, the ideal approach is a joined-up one, where ADHD is considered alongside hormonal health, lifestyle and any coexisting conditions, but unfortunately at the time of writing this we are not in this place or space.

Self-identification and self-accommodation

If you have had a sudden awakening that you may have ADHD or even a new but late diagnosis, the next weeks and months can be deeply transformative on a personal level. You may flit between feeling liberated and disorientated. Everything you have ever known and overcome will now be called into question. The schooling you struggled to reach your potential in, the relationships that didn't work out as you intended, the jobs you loved and lost or struggled to succeed in will now be reflected on and reframed from personal failures to signs of undiagnosed and unsupported ADHD. You may have masked so well over the years that even you didn't recognise it (see Janice's story in Chapter 1). Some women will feel grief and loss, anger and confusion, some will feel empowered and validated, and many of you will fluctuate between all these emotions.

Once you have come to terms with your diagnosis (or likely diagnosis, if you are currently undiagnosed), the next step is to adapt your life to suit your brain. I truly believe that those with ADHD do not struggle all their lives because they have ADHD, they struggle because our society makes them fit into a neurotypical world. I encourage you to not feel bad that your mask has slipped, but to take pleasure in ripping off any mask that remains. By this I mean stop trying to accommodate what other people ask of you, get to know your own strengths and weaknesses and make your life work around them. One positive thing about this period of your life is that perimenopause is often great at helping you care less about what others think, and I encourage you to make the most of this!

Make practical adjustments to your environment, declutter and simplify your surroundings, reframe your self-talk and reset your boundaries to suit you. Seek help for your perimenopause, whether that's HRT, alternatives to HRT or lifestyle changes (see Chapters 2 and 7). You are not stupid, lazy or incapable. You are wired differently and that's ok. In fact, it's more than ok, it's blooming brilliant!

Calling out your inner voice

We all have an inner voice. This is an ongoing stream of thoughts, self-talk and internal running commentary. It comes from a complex mix of our life experiences, our developmental psychology and our cultural conditioning. As children we hear many external voices speak to us and about us, and over time we are likely to internalise these as our self-talk. For some of us these voices can be mostly positive, but for many of you with ADHD they are distinctly negative.

For those with ADHD, your internal voice is quite likely to be highly self-critical, perfectionistic and shaped by past experiences where you have felt like a failure or incapable. Many of you may have been repeatedly told you are 'too much' or 'not enough' which now manifests as negative and highly critical self-talk, poor self-esteem and a lack of self-belief. In fact, some of you will have such low self-esteem because of your inner voice, you will believe that any success you do have is down to luck rather than achievement, even if presented with evidence to the contrary.

A significant number of you will experience rejection sensitive dysphoria (RSD), as discussed in Chapter 3. To recap, this is an intense emotional response to real or perceived criticism or rejection. You may recognise this as the replay you run repeatedly in your mind of a social interaction, whereby you analyse others' tone of voice, facial expressions and the aura or impression they gave you.

For some, this may be so harmful to your wellbeing that you will avoid social interactions altogether for fear of looking stupid or messing up. Another common feature is that of internalised ableism: women may adopt beliefs that their struggles are character flaws, accompanied by negative self-talk such as 'I must try harder' or 'what's wrong with me'. I will say it again: there is nothing wrong with you. ADHD is not a failure or a fault; being forced to live in a neurotypical society when you are neurodivergent is.

Our inner voice reflects what we have absorbed growing up, about who we are and who we should be. This is shaped by our family, our schooling, our cultural and religious interactions, and societal expectations. So many women tell me that years of being told they aren't fit for purpose has taken its toll on their inner monologue, with devastating effects. The great news is your inner voice isn't fixed, and you can change it. The even better news is perimenopause, and midlife generally, is the perfect time to start working on this because if you don't already, you're about to care less about what others think of you! Hold that thought, gather up that perimenopausal sense of liberation and try the following exercise.

Exercise: Changing your inner voice (grab a notepad or your notes app!)

Step 1: Catch the Voice

Take a few minutes to pause and ask: What is my inner voice saying right now?

Don't censor or correct it. Write down exactly what comes up, even if it's mean, rushed, or contradictory.

Some examples women have shared with me:

- 'You're lazy, you never finish anything.'
- 'You should have figured this out by now.'
- 'This is typical – you always drop the ball.'

Step 2: Name the Voice

Now ask yourself: Whose voice is this really? Where did I first hear this sentiment?

You might notice it echoes:

- A parent's impatience
- A teacher's criticism
- A partner's judgement
- A broader cultural script from societal expectations
- Your own expectations of yourself (perfectionist expectations)

Step 3: Talk Back – or Talk Beside

Reframe with compassion:

- Old: 'You're so lazy, you never finish anything.'
- New: 'You've got so much energy and so many great ideas, it's hard not to keep starting new things. It's a gift to be creative and enthusiastic.'

Use your wise self:

Imagine you're speaking to a younger you, or a friend, sister or child with ADHD.

- 'This (e.g. time management) is not your forte, but you have plenty of other skills that many people would long for.'
- 'It's okay to need a list or a timer (or whatever helps you manage). That doesn't make you broken, it makes you human.'

Try humour or metaphor:
- 'Thanks, boring inner voice. You've said your piece. Now let me be me and give the creative brain a chance to speak.'

Step 4: Choose a Phrase to Keep

Get your chosen phrase on a keyring, chain, wallet card or something similar. Return to this when your inner voice gets loud. Here are some examples:

- 'This is a snag, not a failure.'
- 'My brain is different, not defective.'
- 'Having ADHD is not a disadvantage; being forced to live in a neurotypical society is.'
- 'I'm learning to speak to myself kindly.'

In all these steps, the key is you are not trying to bury your unwanted inner voice. Quite the opposite: you are calling it out and telling it that it is seeing things inaccurately. The brain eventually believes what we tell it. Your thinking creates your beliefs, and your beliefs drive your feelings. One of my favourite sayings ever is hanging on my GP consultation wall and it's this:

'If we change the way we look at things, the things we look at change.' By Dr. Wayne Dyer

Helping loved ones understand

I spoke to a patient recently who was incredibly relieved to have been diagnosed in her late 40s with ADHD after lifelong struggles compounded by hormonal flux. She was also incredibly upset, having asked her parents and siblings to watch a documentary on TV that she felt may explain her new diagnosis and how this had translated into her lifelong challenges. They had refused to either watch the documentary or acknowledge her diagnosis and what it meant. She was devastated.

In my experience, the response of loved ones to women seeking a midlife diagnosis of ADHD is as variable as the condition itself. For some of you, your loved ones will be totally on board and supportive, while others – like my patient – may face dismissal and denial. And of course, there's a wide range in between.

Just like your inner voice, there are things you can do to improve the situation, but ultimately this is your time to develop some self-compassion and mould your environment to your neurodivergent brain. Sometimes this involves distancing yourself from situations or people that force you to live neurotypically, at least in the short term.

Having said that, helping your loved ones understand ADHD – especially how it shows up in women – can be a game-changer for supporting relationships, self-esteem and self-development. Here are my eight tips to help them show up for you:

8 Essentials to help loved ones show up for you and your journey

1. Start with the basics

If ever I'm tasked with explaining a new concept to someone, I always begin by assessing their start point. There is so much misinformation and assumption about ADHD, even among medical professionals, that we can't expect our loved ones to know how it shows up, especially in women. Start by asking questions like:

'What does ADHD mean to you? Have you got any thoughts about how it may affect me?'

You may be surprised by the answers in one way or another!

I'd also suggest linking the definition of ADHD to how it affects you personally. Here's an example: 'It's a neurodevelopmental condition that affects attention regulation, impulse control, motivation, memory, emotional regulation, and executive function in the brain. I find I struggle with . . . . . . because of . . . .

The next thing I try to get a handle on when I'm explaining a concept is how someone likes to hear information. Do they like the science, the emotions, the data or the descriptive tales and reflections? It may help, for example, to explain the science behind the genetics and the brain changes (see Chapter 2) that demonstrates tangible evidence of differences (not deficits) in the neurodivergent brain. I understand that sharing all this at once can feel overwhelming. If so, I recommend explaining it in chunks and making notes if you need to, which you could also share with the person you're explaining to.

2. Explain the invisible load

Many women with ADHD are high functioning externally but burning out on the inside. Those around you may have no clue that you've been masking and exhausted for years. It can also mean they struggle to understand why you 'suddenly' think you have ADHD. Of course, this is not sudden for you, who have been carrying these challenges your whole life. Most people have no clue that ADHD can suddenly worsen and become visible in perimenopause and menopause (or with any hormonal change).

Help them see:

- This isn't a new thing; it's been missed for years.
- You're not lazy; you're navigating constant mental noise.
- Simple tasks can feel like climbing a mountain when executive function is low.
- Emotional regulation can be harder due to rejection sensitive dysphoria, brain differences and the effect of fluctuating hormones on the brain in perimenopause (see Chapters 2 and 3).

3. **Use analogies and visuals**

It may help to have some analogies to hand to help convey how you feel.

For example: 'It's like having 50 browser tabs open, all playing sound at once, and being expected to focus on one calmly.'

You might also want to share:

- A short YouTube video (e.g. the 'How to ADHD' channel)
- A comic or infographic (e.g. those by Dani Donovan)
- A podcast episode or TED talk (e.g. 'Is it ADHD or life? A Couple's Perspective' from the *ADHD or Life?* podcast)
- A website with useful resources (e.g. ADHD UK)

4. Talk about gender differences in ADHD

One of the biggest misconceptions about ADHD is that you must be impulsive and hyperactive. It may help for you to explain that ADHD in women is often:

- Internalised hyperactivity (overthinking, anxiety, perfectionism)
- Missed due to masking and social conditioning
- Associated with guilt, shame and late diagnosis

Identifying that most women are diagnosed later in life helps to frame the fact this is a common missed diagnosis, not a midlife crisis or a decision you've just taken.

5. Ask for what you need, don't expect them to know

People often want to help but don't know how and sometimes don't want to ask, especially if they too have spent years avoiding outbursts by trying not to trigger your RSD! It is worth recognising that while living with ADHD for many years can be destructive, living with someone you love who has ADHD can also be challenging at times. Set some boundaries about what is ok to ask for and suggest clarity on both sides.
Examples:

- 'It helps when you text me the day before we meet.'
- 'When I zone out, I'm not being rude; it helps if you gently check in.'
- 'Please don't say "just make a list"; I usually have 20 lists already. It helps if you can remind me without judgement.'
- 'When I'm feeling criticised, telling me I'm over-reacting then makes me feel stupid – please just take a step back.'
- 'Sometimes I need a hug, and sometimes I need space; neither is a reflection on you, but it really

helps if I can let you know which one I need in a given moment.'

- 'You probably already know I'm menopausal and that this can make my moods swing, but the hormones changing can also impact the parts of my brain that are already affected by ADHD and this makes matters worse on all fronts.'

6. Be real about the emotions

ADHD can bring:

- Guilt over not doing 'simple' things
- Fear of disappointing others
- Burnout from masking
- Low self-esteem

Perimenopause and menopause can bring:

- Loss of confidence
- Changing body image
- Loss of self and identity
- Grief and regret

I find this a useful phrase that can be adapted to your own emotions and reasons:

'I carry a lot of shame about not being consistent. When I feel safe and understood, I can show up more fully.'

This phrase can also be a powerful way of expressing your loss of self:

'I feel like I don't know who I am anymore or who I'm meant to be. When you help me identify parts of myself I used to know, this helps my confidence and wellbeing.'

Tell them how they can help you feel safe and understood because, honestly, as a parent of a child with inattentive ADHD and RSD, I don't always know. It doesn't mean I don't want to be there or support them – but sometimes I need help to understand how.

7. **Set boundaries, celebrate strengths and adjust for weaknesses**

Understanding ADHD isn't about excusing everything as ADHD. It's about setting healthy expectations, and recognising your strengths and weaknesses so you and those around you can adjust to them. Some of the key strengths of those with ADHD can include:

- Creativity
- Deep empathy
- Hyperfocus on passions
- Ability to problem-solve in nonlinear ways

Finding roles that play to these strengths in your personal and work life can be liberating. Finding ways with your loved ones to overcome common weaknesses such as time blindness and poor working memory can be a game-changer for everyone and reduce unnecessary conflict. At the back of this book, you will also find several resources you may want to share with loved ones (see page 209).

TL;DR – Chapter 6: Diagnosis or Self-Identifying your ADHD in Perimenopause or Menopause

In this chapter, we've explored the rollercoaster of potentially seeking a diagnosis for ADHD while navigating perimenopause and menopause in midlife. We've looked at ways to change your inner voice to support you, and how to help loved ones do the same. In the next chapter, we will explore hormonal therapy and the potential effects of this for those with ADHD.

The Pros and Cons of Formal ADHD Diagnosis in Midlife

Pros:

- Provides clarity and self-understanding for lifelong struggles.
- Can validate your experiences, especially as hormones shift in perimenopause/menopause.
- Enables access to ADHD-specific medications, therapies and workplace accommodations.
- May help you manage menopause more effectively through joined-up care.
- Offers the chance for self-acceptance and reframing past challenges.

Cons:

- Diagnosis during hormonal transition can cause confusion (is it ADHD or hormones?).
- Grief and regret over missed opportunities and late recognition.
- ADHD medications may be harder to tolerate in menopause (e.g. due to sleep issues, CVD risks).
- No unified approach currently exists to assess both ADHD and menopause together.

Self-Identification and Self-Accommodation

- Not everyone needs a formal diagnosis; self-identification can be transformative.
- Focus on adapting your life to suit your brain, not the other way around.
- Let go of the mask. Simplify your life. Work with your strengths.
- You're not lazy or broken, you're wired differently and that's brilliant.

Finding Your Own Language

- ADHD often leads to harsh inner self-talk formed from years of criticism.
- Perimenopause can amplify feelings of loss, confusion and RSD (rejection sensitive dysphoria).
- Learn to recognise, name and reframe your inner voice with compassion.
- Change your internal narrative to change your emotional reality.

Helping Loved Ones Understand

1. Start with the basics; explain ADHD, especially how it shows up in women.
2. Discuss the invisible load; show them the masking and exhaustion.
3. Explain gender differences, masking, internalisation, late diagnosis.
4. Ask for specific support; don't expect them to just know what you need.
5. Be open about emotions; guilt, burnout, identity loss are real.

Diagnosis is helpful, but not essential – many find empowerment through self-understanding. Speak kindly to yourself. Educate others but protect your energy and boundaries.

Focus on fitting your world to your brain, not vice versa.

Chapter 7
Hormones, HRT, ADHD Medication and Cognition Support

Topics covered in this chapter:

- HRT: the basics
- HRT and ADHD: what we know we know (and what we don't yet know)
- Lifestyle and holistic approaches to ADHD and perimenopausal management
- ADHD medication overview: what you need to know
- Cognitive shifts in ADHD and perimenopause: what's happening and how to cope

Hopefully by this point in the book you have clarity on some of the key issues it covers: what neurodivergence is (specifically ADHD), how to recognise it in yourself, and how the hormonal changes in perimenopause and menopause can impact our hormones and in turn our chemical brain messengers, looping back to unmask your ADHD.

In this chapter we will look more closely at hormone replacement therapy (HRT), the first-line treatment for perimenopause and menopause in all current guidance globally. I will talk you through (in simplistic terms) what HRT is, when and why you may be given it, in what form, and the potential pros and cons of this. Finally, we will close this chapter looking at what we know and don't know about the use of HRT in ADHD, and what other approaches may help with your perimenopausal ADHD alongside or instead of ADHD medication.

Please note, there is some discussion at the moment about changing the terminology from hormone replacement therapy (HRT) to menopause hormone treatment (MHT). At the time of writing, HRT is the commonly used name for this treatment, so it is the term I have used throughout this book.

HRT: the basics

In Chapter 5 I talked about the difficulties you may face in getting timely and informative menopause care from your GP and what you can, in my opinion, realistically expect. Like most things in medicine and science, our understanding of common issues and their management is constantly shifting, and menopause and HRT are no exception.

During my time as a doctor, I have seen huge shifts in how we use and view the benefits and risks of HRT. When I first became a GP many years ago, oral HRT was standard, and patches only prescribed in very few select cases (usually due to patient preference). We typically only saw women presenting for HRT when they were very clearly of menopausal age and stage of life (around 50) and of course many women didn't attend at all. We were, in my opinion, fixated on the classic symptoms of hot flushes, night sweats and mood changes. I shudder to think how many midlife women I saw in whom I didn't even consider hormonal changes when they were presenting with a multitude of other symptoms such as aches and pains and brain fog. Finally, we talked a lot about 'substantial risks' associated with HRT (especially that of breast cancer) and very little about the potential long-term benefits of HRT. The Million Women Study and similar early research in the early 2000s caused significant harm to women's and clinicians' confidence in hormone replacement therapy (HRT). These studies suggested a strong link between HRT and breast cancer, leading to widespread fear and a sharp decline in use almost overnight. However, we now know that these findings were overstated and have since been substantially reinterpreted. Later, more robust analyses showed that the increased breast cancer risk associated with HRT is much smaller than originally reported, and in fact is lower than the risks linked to common lifestyle factors such as drinking alcohol, being overweight and physical inactivity in most women. Importantly, many types of HRT used today are more physiologically aligned with women's natural hormones (known as body-identical) and appear to carry a lower risk profile. While HRT is not entirely without risk, our current understanding is far more balanced, allowing women and clinicians to make informed, confident choices based on accurate evidence and discussion of both the risks and benefits.

Hormone replacement therapy (HRT) is a hormonal treatment that supports a woman's own underlying oestrogen and progesterone hormones as they fluctuate in the transition phase of perimenopause and ultimately decrease in menopause. This can be with either body-identical progesterone or synthetic versions (called progestins). You can read more about this on page 154. Women who experience post-surgical menopause due to removal of the ovaries before the age of 50 usually have a significantly quicker decline in hormones and often need extra hormonal support to help with function and protecting the bones, heart and brain from premature and rapid hormone loss.

In time, your body will hopefully reset to the new lower hormone levels, but getting to that point can be a challenging journey for some women and, consequently, some choose to stay on HRT long-term (and providing they are regularly risk assessed and reviewed, guidance now supports this view). HRT has been shown to help with symptoms including hot flushes, poor sleep, mood changes and vaginal dryness, and we now know it may also help protect bone, heart and possibly brain health in the longer term. HRT comes in different forms, such as tablets, patches, gels and sprays and the choice of how to take HRT often depends on personal preference, medical history, convenience and how your body responds. There is no 'one size fits all' approach.

If you have had a total hysterectomy and have no womb tissue left, then you can have oestrogen-only HRT, but most women require combined HRT (oestrogen and progesterone) for added protection. Womb (endometrial) tissue can become overactive if oestrogen is used without progesterone and over time, this can lead to womb (endometrial) cancer. If you had a hysterectomy due to endometriosis (womb tissue locating itself where it shouldn't be) then you may still need combined HRT in case of residual womb lining tissue somewhere.

If you are perimenopausal, still have periods or are within 12 months of your last period, you will usually start with sequential HRT. Sequential HRT means the hormones oestrogen and progesterone are given in a sequence; oestrogen all the time and progesterone for part of the month (12–14 days) to mimic your underlying natural hormone cycle. You will likely still have a bleed, although this may lessen as you move closer towards menopause.

As already noted, we are now seeing women in clinical practice who are much younger and earlier into their perimenopause journey than in previous years. I do not think women are experiencing perimenopause earlier by and large, but I do suspect we have got better at recognising it and empowering women to not put up with it. Some clinicians may turn to the combined contraceptive pill to help with perimenopausal symptoms in younger women who also need contraception and/or regulation of their cycles. It may feel more familiar or appropriate to some clinicians as we navigate this changing picture of how women present and when. Theoretically, you can have the combined contraceptive pill up to the age of 50 with appropriate annual review of the risks and benefits and providing there are no factors that make taking the combined pill unsafe (for example if you are a smoker, have high blood pressure, or suffer from migraines with aura). The oestrogen in the combined contraceptive pill will likely help early perimenopause symptoms but the doses of hormones in the combined contraceptive pill can be in excess and more synthetic in nature than those in HRT, meaning the risks of blood clots and so on can be higher and may not be tolerated as well. In my experience, it can be much harder for a woman with underlying neurodivergence to find a contraceptive that she tolerates well. My advice is to keep an open mind but, for most women, personally, I would opt for a trial of HRT if hormones deemed medically safe and appropriate after individual assessment.

If you are post-menopausal and haven't had a bleed for 12 months or more (or over the age of 54, if on contraception that means you are unsure when your last period was), you will require continuous HRT. Continuous combined HRT combines both hormones (oestrogen and progesterone) continuously, every day, and usually does not create a bleed (although this can take 3–6 months to fully settle). At some point in your transition to menopause you will require a shift from sequential to continuous therapy to protect your womb lining. It can be difficult to know when to make this shift.

These days, many women are offered transdermal HRT (hormones through the skin as a patch, gel or spray) rather than tablets (although these are still available and suit some women well). This is because taking oestrogen through the skin avoids the liver, so it doesn't raise the risk of blood clots or strokes in the same way tablets can, and it often produces a steadier hormone level. It is also better suited for women who have migraines, higher blood pressure, or other health risks.

HRT preparations at a glance
Transdermal: through the skin, comes in the form of a gel, patch or spray
Oral: taken as a tablet or capsule
Combined: oestrogen and progesterone
Sequential: oestrogen taken every day and progesterone at least 12–14 days per month
Continuous: oestrogen and progesterone taken every day

Nothing in life is without risk, least of all medication, but those risks need to be tailored to you as an individual and your circumstances. It is also important for risks to be placed in perspective; having a BMI of 30 or above or drinking alcohol on a regular basis may elevate your risk of breast cancer more than the use of combined HRT for most women. For many women, the benefits of symptom relief, bone protection and improved quality of life far outweigh these relatively small risks. Individual baseline risk, type of progestogen, duration of HRT use and other personalised factors are important to consider. In Chapter 2, you can find information about the potential alternatives to HRT for perimenopause, such as SSRIs and gabapentin.

HRT and ADHD: what we know (and what we don't yet know)

The fact that hormones have an impact on the female brain is basic neuroscience. The rest of the story, like most things that affect women in medicine, is seriously underfunded and under-researched. As a result, at lot of what we know or do practically for women with ADHD in perimenopause is based on theory and anecdote, not evidence. This doesn't make it necessarily wrong, but it does leave us with some uncertainty. It also makes it harder to roll out any best practice to clinicians, which compounds the problem of women being dismissed. Most people don't want to know about problems they can't fix, and some clinicians are no exception to this. Guidance is usually based on some form of evidence-based practice and at the present time we have very little.

Here are some key facts and theory about female hormones and the brain that we have actual evidence for when considering the use of HRT in ADHD:

- Oestrogen and dopamine are closely linked, as discussed at length in Chapter 2. Oestrogen enhances dopamine function (as well as other key chemical messengers), dopamine release, and receptor availability and sensitivity (how well circulating dopamine can be used by the brain). Dopamine regulation is key in ADHD.
- Progesterone can have a dampening effect on dopamine activity. This can modestly impair attention, motivation and mood. Many women report cyclical worsening of ADHD symptoms in the luteal phase of the menstrual cycle (the second half, just before a period when your progesterone is high and oestrogen is low). For many women, the progesterone breakdown product (called allopregnanolone) acting on GABA-A receptors in the brain has a calming effect. However, neurodivergent women (evidence currently strongest for those with ADHD) can often experience an altered response to these receptors, potentially leading to increased irritability and anxiety. Women with ADHD also seem to have a higher incidence of PMDD and PMS due to this progesterone sensitivity.
- There is growing evidence that neurodivergent

women can experience atypical brain responses to sex hormones (especially oestrogen and progesterone, the latter of which we discussed in the last bullet point). These differences are likely linked to variations in brain receptors and the action of any breakdown products of the hormones. Sadly, research is still very limited and what few studies are available are not widely acknowledged yet.

- ADHD symptoms often worsen at perimenopause and menopause, when oestrogen fluctuates then declines (see Chapter 2). There are other key times relating to oestrogen decline when ADHD may worsen, such as post-pregnancy, demonstrating this link.
- Many women with ADHD are diagnosed late, or misdiagnosed, often after hormonal shifts (such as perimenopause) unmask symptoms.
- We now think that starting HRT early in your perimenopause (before age 60 or within 10 years of menopause) may be protective to our brain cells, and we know oestrogen is neuroprotective (see Chapter 4). This applies broadly to women at this stage of life, not just those with ADHD.

There are other considerations that we know to be true based on anecdotal evidence and experience. For example, we know from many women with ADHD that HRT has had a positive effect on their cognition (thinking), attention, and executive function by supporting predominantly dopamine (plus other chemical messenger) pathways. There are some potential downsides; if you have ADHD, taking HRT daily may be tricky to remember and be consistent with, and if you are also taking stimulant medication the overlapping possible cardiovascular risks may need some consideration, although lots of women take both with good effect.

Sadly, there is still a lot we don't know or have evidence for around the topic of HRT in ADHD. At the time of writing there are no 'gold standard' randomised controlled trials (RCTs) that directly study the effects of HRT on those with ADHD and its symptoms. Most of what we know comes from listening to women who have tried it, talking to clinicians who have prescribed it and extending the theory of oestrogen and other hormones on the brain into real life practice.

As a result, there is a lot we don't yet know – such as whether transdermal or oral HRT works best in women with ADHD and whether women with ADHD do better with body-identical or synthetic progestogen, and at what dose. The progestogen element is poorly understood. Not all progestogens are equal in any woman, however neurotypical or divergent you are. All women appear to respond uniquely to this hormone, but we think ADHD can compound this. Progestogen is a recognised medical term that refers to any hormone with progesterone-like activity, including both natural progesterone (identical to the hormone our bodies produce) and synthetic versions (man-made and structurally different from our own body's progesterone), often called pro-gestins. While this terminology has existed in medicine for some time, the conversation about different progestogens and how women experience them is increasingly being led by women themselves, sometimes ahead of formal clinical discussion. Currently, there is limited evidence to guide our understanding of which women respond best to which type of progestogen, or why, and this is reflected in the lack of clear guidance in standard clinical practice (and often a resulting lack of discussion around the same). It's important to remember that struggling with one preparation does not necessarily predict your response to another, whether it's a different type, dose or route of administration. The best approach is to work collaboratively with your GP (or meno-pause clinician), armed with good information, patience and an open mindset, recognising that finding the right option may take some trial and adjustment and that this process is a normal and valid part of personalised care.

- Progesterone: the hormone your body naturally produces
- Micronised progesterone: also known as body-identical, because it has the same structure as the hormone made by your ovaries (common brand names include Utrogestan and Gepretix)
- Progestogen: this is the broad umbrella term that includes all forms of hormone that act like progesterone in the body; body-identical or synthetic
- Progestin: the man-made and structurally different, synthetic versions of progestogen – these vary in structure and effect (common drug names include norethisterone and levonorgestrel).

In my experience, inability to tolerate the progestogen component of HRT is one of the key reasons why women and clinicians give up on it. This can show up as increased anxiety, agitation, mood swings, bloating and breast tenderness, among other symptoms. I am labouring this point because not all clinicians may be fully aware of the extent to which a change in progestogen (type or route of administration) may help you and I want to empower you to have this discussion if needed. Some women cannot or do not want to take HRT from the outset and some women try HRT and stop it as they don't like it. In my opinion, too many women don't have HRT because they are given incorrect advice or aren't supported to tweak the route, dose and/or type for long enough to feel better.

Below, I highlight several reasons why every single woman may vary in her response to progestogen type, dose and route. I'm not here to drown you in science, but I want you to appreciate just how nuanced our bodies' responses to any given progestogen are, and how we can't expect a standard response in anyone.

Here's what we know about why all women may respond differently to the same progestogen (you can skip this bit if you don't want the science):

Hormone receptor sensitivity

Progesterone receptors (PR-A and PR-B that attach to progesterone to make it work) vary in number and responsiveness between individuals. Some women may have lower receptor sensitivity or receptors that don't respond well, reducing their effectiveness. Even if enough progesterone is present in the blood stream, it may not be working like it should as the body can't accept it.

Genetics

Gene variants can affect how a progestogen is broken down (metabolised) or how receptors function. Differences in the PGR gene (which codes for the progesterone receptor) or in CYP enzymes (which metabolise hormones) may change treatment response.

Route of administration

Oral, transdermal, and vaginal progestogens all have different bioavailability (how much is useable when broken down in the body) and effects. For example, oral micronised progesterone is metabolised in the liver and can have sedative effects, which some women tolerate better than others.

Brain receptor response

Progestogen breakdown products interact with GABA-A receptors in the brain. These often have calming or mood-modulating effects, but for some people (particularly neurodivergent women), they can also worsen anxiety, irritability, low mood, or fatigue depending on brain chemistry (as detailed in Chapter 2). Some synthetic progestins cannot be converted into breakdown products that have this neuro-calming effect.

Metabolic and liver function

The liver plays a key role in hormone metabolism. Differences in liver enzyme activity, body weight, or potentially gut microbiome (ongoing research) can affect how much active progesterone circulates and how long it stays active if given orally.

Underlying conditions

Conditions like premenstrual dysphoric disorder (PMDD), endometriosis, polycystic ovary syndrome (PCOS), perimenopause, or thyroid issues may influence how well progestogens work (or rather how women experience and tolerate them). For example, in premenstrual dysphoric disorder (PMDD), there's often an altered GABA-A receptor response to normal progesterone fluctuations. Ordinarily, as progesterone rises before a period is due, the breakdown products of progesterone (allopregnanolone) act on GABA-A receptors to produce a calming, mood-stabilising effect. In women with PMDD, however, altered receptor functioning and brain circuits can mean the opposite can happen, causing irritability, anxiety, anger and low or erratic mood.

Psychological and environmental factors

Stress levels, trauma history and mental health status can all affect the body's hormonal response and therefore how it interacts with other hormones that are taken in (called the HPA axis). This may be why you can be fine with one progestogen at a certain stage in your life and completely overwhelmed by it several years later.

Forms of progestogen

There is a wide scope of HRT products containing a whole host of progestogens, from synthetic to body-identical versions. Conversely, many contraceptives have mainly synthetic progestins.

Body-identical (micronised) progesterone tends to be better tolerated by some women than synthetic progestins like medroxyprogesterone or norethisterone. It makes sense that synthetic (man-made) hormone products that are chemically different to the ones our bodies make ourselves can be harder to get on with. It is important to note, however, that this is not the case for all women, and some do much better with synthetic progestins, probably for the reasons above.

The bottom line is that where progestogens are concerned, there is no 'one size fits all' for any woman. Women with ADHD can react very badly to a progestogen they don't tolerate, whether in the form of HRT or contraception. We need to understand this better on a practical level to provide the right regime and support. Currently it is very much guesswork with trial and error, and unfortunately women suffer in the process. My advice, as above, is to not suffer in silence; I very much hope the information provided here will inform, enable and most of all empower you to go back to your doctor to discuss this situation further and the possibility of trialling a different progestogen type or route.

Progesterone intolerance

I have come across so many women who admit to missing doses or completely omitting the progestogen element of their HRT when it is given as two separate hormones (e.g. an oestrogen patch with progesterone tablets to take for half the month). Many people cite intolerable side effects as the reason for this. Please do not take your oestrogen patch, gel or spray without a form of progestogen if it has been prescribed to you. I cannot stress enough how important this is. Taking less than the recommended 12–14 days per month of a progestogen in a sequential HRT regime over just a few months can lead to womb tissue and cell changes that can ultimately and over time increase your risk of womb (endometrial) cancer. If you aren't getting on with the progestogen element of your HRT, it's time to change the type or route.

It is worth noting that using micronised progesterone vaginally in the same dose and form as you would orally is off licence in the UK (as in, outside the terms of its official marketing authorisation), and, particularly at higher doses of oestrogen, may be a less robust and less evidenced way of protecting your womb lining. This route of administration is not recommended routinely over licensed therapies. However, this method is currently acknowledged within guidance at the time of writing when oral progestogen is not tolerated. I hope going to your GP armed with the information provided within this chapter will help you feel empowered to discuss alternative options.

Starting HRT for any woman is a journey, not a destination. There is often a little bit of tweaking that needs to occur and some of you will need a complete chop and change to find the HRT that works well for you.

Lack of long-term data

Another uncertainty in what we know and don't know around ADHD and the perimenopause is the lack of long-term outcome data. As things stand, there is no data on long-term outcomes, such as cognition and cardiovascular risk, in women with ADHD who are using HRT. These risks have been studied at length in the general population over recent years with mainly reassuring results, but now we need to recognise the subset of women with ADHD. ADHD is already associated with increased cardiovascular and metabolic risks to some extent, so when HRT is involved, we could anticipate that women may require individual risk assessment alongside guidance which would need to be based on research that we don't have yet.

The link between ADHD and increased cardiovascular and metabolic risks is increasingly recognised in research, particularly in adults and especially in women, where underdiagnosis may delay treatment and lifestyle interventions.

- ADHD is a neurodevelopmental condition that affects impulse control, emotional regulation, motivation and self-management, all of which play a major role in long-term physical health outcomes.
- People with ADHD are statistically more likely to have irregular eating habits (skipping meals, binge eating, preference for ultra-processed or sugary foods), struggle with sleep disorders (insomnia, delayed sleep phase, poor sleep hygiene), smoke or use substances while chasing dopamine, have higher rates of disordered eating, particularly binge-eating and emotional eating, and experience anxiety and/or depression.

- As a result of other factors, those with ADHD may be potentially more likely to have obesity, insulin resistance, high blood pressure and cholesterol; all these factors impact heart health and long-term risk of heart attacks and stroke.
- Dopamine dysregulation, a central aspect of ADHD, also plays a role in appetite control, reward processing and impulse regulation. Some research suggests altered cortisol levels and chronic low-grade inflammation in people with ADHD, leading to poorer cardiac health. There's also evidence of autonomic nervous system dysregulation (the part of our nervous system responsible for our bodily functions we don't knowingly control), which may influence heart rate variability and stress responses.
- Most ADHD medication is stimulant based (e.g. methylphenidate, lisdexamfetamine). Stimulant medication can slightly increase heart rate and blood pressure. In most people, this is mild and not clinically significant but for those with pre-existing heart conditions, monitoring is important (or in some cases avoid). Having said this, treatment of ADHD often improves self-regulation, allowing for better lifestyle habits, weight control and lower long-term risk. Studies suggest that untreated ADHD may carry greater long-term cardiovascular risk than ADHD treated with stimulant-based medications.

It would make good sense medically to routinely screen those with ADHD for things like blood pressure, blood sugar and cholesterol. We do this as a matter of course for many conditions and age groups, yet we do not routinely review those with ADHD.

What we need to see happen:

- Gold-standard research: RCTs (randomised controlled trials) comparing ADHD symptom changes with and without HRT.
- Studies of using HRT stratified by age, menopausal stage and neurodivergent profile.
- Research into how different progestogens affect the ADHD brain and the potential resultant side effect profiles (more specifically, their effects on dopamine regulation).
- A deeper understanding of how women with ADHD may respond to hormones and what to do to manage it.
- Guidance on how best to manage women in peri-menopause with ADHD.

For now, we need women like you to feel empowered enough to step forward for help. To be seen and listened to. The use of HRT in women with ADHD may not be as evidence-based as we would like but it certainly seems to help stabilise some women, especially if you can stick with the journey of getting the right form of HRT for you. I hope that this chapter has, so far, given you some confidence to do just that.

Lifestyle and holistic approaches to ADHD and perimenopausal management

For many of you, getting diagnosed will be a very difficult, lengthy and emotional process. Getting medicated may be something you are unsure of, don't want to venture into or can't do medically or practically. With or without medication, there are several lifestyle tweaks that may help support your ADHD brain during perimenopause or menopause. Remember, your brain isn't faulty or failing, you just haven't always known the best ways to maximise its potential. Some of the following information may help.

Nutrition

Your ADHD brain will have altered dopamine and other chemical messenger regulation. Nutrition can influence the availability of chemical messengers and inflammation. Blood sugar fluctuations, particularly rapid blood sugar spikes and crashes, can make inattention, hyperactivity and irritability worse.

High protein, low glycaemic index (GI)

Evidence for nutrition-based strategies are somewhat limited, but we do know that high protein diets and meals with a lower glycaemic index (foods that cause a slower, more gradual rise in blood sugar levels after eating) may help stabilise your blood sugar and in theory support chemical messenger (such as dopamine) supply, function and stability.

Low GI foods:

Fruits: apples, berries, pears, oranges
Vegetables: carrots, broccoli, peppers, tomatoes
Legumes: lentils, chickpeas, beans
Grains: oats, barley, quinoa
Dairy: skimmed milk, plain yoghurt

High GI foods:

Grains: white bread, white rice
Sugary drinks: juice, fizzy drinks
Snacks: most processed snack foods such as crisps, sweets and pastries

High protein foods:

Lean meats and poultry: beef, lamb, pork, chicken, turkey
Fish: salmon, tuna, crab
Eggs and dairy: milk, yoghurt, cheese

Legumes: lentils, beans, chickpeas, tofu
Nuts and seeds: almonds, pumpkin seeds, peanuts

Low protein foods
Fruits: apples, bananas, peaches, berries
Vegetables: tomatoes, peppers, broccoli
Grains: rice, pasta, oats, bread

Omega-3 fatty acids
Omega-3 fatty acids (EPA > DHA; see below) may improve attention and mood. Evidence is modest but growing to support the use of omega-3 supplements. In clinical trials doses of 500–1,000mg EPA per day have shown the most benefit and having a higher ratio of EPA to DHA has been shown to be more effective than DHA alone or equal amounts of both. DHA has less consistent benefits in treating core ADHD symptoms but is still important for overall brain health. If you are choosing a supplement, look for one with a high EPA content compared to DHA content – for example: 750mg EPA to 250mg DHA.

EPA (eicosapentaenoic acid): mainly supports heart health and reduces inflammation and appears most consistently linked to improvement in ADHD symptoms.

DHA (docosahexaenoic acid): essential for brain function and eye health. May support working memory and emotional regulation though evidence is less consistent than for EPA.

Foods rich in omega-3: mackerel, salmon, sardines, anchovies, herring

Non-fish options: chia seeds, flaxseeds, walnuts, hemp seeds. These don't contain EPA or DHA but they do contain ALA which can be converted (though not very well) to EPA and DHA.

Other vitamins

Iron, zinc, magnesium and vitamin D are often lower in people with ADHD. Topping these up may help overall brain function.

Top tip: Limit alcohol, excess caffeine, sugar, ultra-processed foods (they exacerbate mood swings and impulsivity).

Gut microbiome

In Chapter 4 we discussed the growing body of research, evidence and support for developing and maintaining a healthy gut microbiome. A healthy gut microbiome can support our immune function, improve mental health and significantly reduce disease. We also explored how the estrobolome within the microbiome can recycle oestrogen and support hormone instability. To maximise this, aim to eat more than 30 plant foods a week, 30g of fibre per day and limit ultra-processed foods, alcohol and unnecessary anti-biotics (by this, I mean antibiotics that are prescribed or taken without clear evidence of bacterial infection).

Movement and exercise

We discussed the power of movement in Chapter 4, but it is so important in perimenopause and ADHD that I couldn't leave it out here. Regular exercise increases dopamine, norepinephrine and serotonin – the same chemical messengers targeted by stimulant medication for your ADHD.

We also know that physical activity improves executive function (thinking and planning), impulse control and mood. Movement can also reduce anxiety, depression and irritability. It is also vitally important in perimenopause to support bone and metabolic health. The hardest part of any exercise regime is getting started. You may find this more of a challenge with ADHD if transitioning from another task or getting distracted.

My advice is not to overwhelm yourself. Pick something you enjoy; any movement is better than none. Start with short episodes and work up to longer and more frequent sessions. Build this into your daily plans, using strategies for time management and technology (apps, alarms and so on) to help you maintain the new routine as discussed in Chapter 3. Here is a suggested exercise plan to begin with:

- **30 minutes most days**: brisk walking, cycling, swimming.
- **Strength training twice a week**: essential in midlife for metabolism, cognition and bone health.
- **Gentler options during burnout**: yoga, Pilates, tai chi (especially during heavy periods or fatigue).
- **Make it ADHD-friendly**: music, outdoor settings, classes, buddy systems.

Sleep

Both perimenopause and ADHD can affect your sleep. As we discovered in Chapter 4, ADHD is strongly associated with the disruption of your circadian rhythm (internal body clock) and delayed sleep phase. Sleep deprivation worsens attention, memory and emotional regulation in everyone, but particularly if you have ADHD. Chapter 4 explores how you can improve your sleep struggles and sleep hygiene. As a GP of many years, I know this is often easy for me to say and hard for you to do, but the first step is acknowledging and accepting that enough sleep is crucial for your ADHD brain to reach its potential, even more so when you are also in perimenopause or menopause.

Mindfulness and stress reduction

We know that mindfulness and meditation can reduce emotional reactivity, regulate your nervous system and improve attention. Stress increases your cortisol level and worsens executive differences and impulsivity. How many times have you felt unable to think straight when worked up or stressed? Your brain literally stops functioning as it should. Hormonal fluctuations can also significantly add to this. Try mindfulness, meditation, breathwork and time in nature to reduce your baseline stress levels and improve your focus. Meditation can be extremely difficult to master with ADHD due to restlessness, difficulty sustaining attention and the mind wandering, often leading to a sense of failure. It can be extremely beneficial for ADHD and perimenopause/menopause but must be adapted with practical approaches for many of you with ADHD.

Start small, just 1–3 minutes at first, and build up slowly. You could consider using guided meditations through apps like Headspace or Insight Timer to hold your attention. Walking meditations, yoga or even mindful stretching can be easier than sitting still. ADHD brains benefit from engaging more than one sense; using sensory cues like sound, breath or touch can help you focus to meditate. A quick tip: try zoning out and practising deep breathing while holding a warm drink for just 1–3 minutes on a regular basis.

With regular practice, meditation can improve attention, reduce emotional reactivity, improve impulse control and enhance sleep by reducing anxiety. Don't expect this practice to be easy but I am confident that you will find it worthwhile when you get there.

Structure, routines and environment

ADHD is a disorder of self-regulation; not a lack of knowing *what* to do, but trouble doing it consistently. Find tools that help you to be consistent such as planners, timers, white-boards and anything that externalises what's in your brain. As discussed in Chapter 3, I recommend you minimise clutter, automate what you can and preplan to minimise decision fatigue. I will never tire of reminding you that your brain is not faulty or failing, you just perhaps haven't known how to get the most out of it for so long.

Connection and support

Adults with ADHD often struggle with shame, rejection sensitivity dysphoria (RSD) and social anxiety. Losing your sense of self, confidence and coping with changing body image can add to this in perimenopause. Staying sociable and supported really helps, although it can at times feel overstimulating and overwhelming. Go at your own pace and know that you don't have to conform to other people's norm.

Midlife often brings identity shifts, caregiving burdens and career transitions. Many women in this stage of life experience burnout and a sense of 'losing themselves'. Avoid environments or people that trigger shame or comparison. Try to surround yourself with people who affirm who you are, lift you up and push you on.

Alternative therapies

Evidence for the efficacy of treatments such as acupuncture and herbal supplements like rhodiola, bacopa, ginkgo and CBD are limited, although you may see them mentioned in some ADHD forums and resources. Similarly, menopause guidance advises caution around herbal remedies and plant-derived compounds due to limited evidence and potential lack of regulation. Some of these herbal menopause supplements contain phytoestrogens; plant compounds that can bind to oestrogen receptors and mimic oestrogen. While this may help some symptoms, some women may wish to or need to avoid oestrogen, and the dose, purity and consistency of ingredients can vary widely. They can also potentially interact with prescribed medication. Most supplements are not regulated as medicines and come under a separate category of food supplements, which means they do not have to meet the strict criteria that medicines do. For this reason, you will find many clinicians are reluctant to recommend such alternative therapies.

Cheat sheet for initial self-help support

Nutrition	High-protein breakfast, reduce processed and high sugar foods. Increase intake of plant foods and fibre, omega 3s and lower GI foods.
Exercise	15–30 minutes movement (walk, yoga, run, stretch) every other day.
Sleep	Wind-down routine: bath, screen down, read, consistent sleep and wake times.
Environment	Declutter and simplify.
Structure	Use planners, whiteboards and other tools. Set 3 daily priorities.
Mindfulness	1–3 minutes daily breathwork or grounding practice.
Connection	Touch base with a friend or support group for ADHD support. Avoid people who don't align with your newfound freedom of mind and spirit.

With the right supports, women can transform overwhelm into clarity. Slow and steady really does win this race.

ADHD medication overview: what you need to know

Medication for ADHD has its benefits. It is often the first-line medical treatment for moderate-to-severe ADHD in adults because it can significantly improve:

- Focus and concentration
- Impulse control
- Emotional regulation
- Task initiation and follow-through

It isn't right for everyone, and not everyone wants to be medicated, and this too is perfectly ok. Not being medicated does not mean your ADHD is 'not that bad', nor does it mean you are not willing to help yourself. It is a personal choice. There are plenty of other ways you can manage your ADHD.

As with all medications, there are some people who will find them more beneficial than others from the outset. Medication is most likely to help adults who:

- Have moderate to severe symptoms that impact daily life, work, relationships, or health
- Struggle with executive function (getting started, switching tasks, focus, organising)
- Experience emotional dysregulation or frequent overwhelm
- Are willing and able to engage in ongoing review and monitoring
- Don't have unmanaged cardiovascular conditions or substance misuse concerns

Situations where stimulant medication may not be suitable or require caution include:

- Uncontrolled high blood pressure, heart disease or

family history of sudden cardiac death in a young family member
- History of psychosis, mania, or bipolar disorder (requires specialist input)
- Pregnant or trying to conceive; stimulant use in pregnancy is a risk–benefit decision: can potentially be used with caution after discussion/ assessment
- History of substance misuse; UK stimulant medications are controlled drugs
- Highly anxious or overstimulated; may find stimulants worsen symptoms initially
- Other medications that may interact.

If you are considering medication and have any of these conditions or medical history, you may be suitable for non-stimulant medication or you may need to avoid medication for your ADHD altogether.

ADHD medication for those who are deemed suitable will eventually help about 70–80 per cent of people. If the dose is too low or too high, or a particular medication is not tolerated well, adjustments likely need to be made. For most people, medication is not a cure-all, but it can make good headway towards a greater sense of clarity for the right individuals.

Types of ADHD medication

Stimulants (first-line treatment in adults with ADHD)

Stimulants act by increasing dopamine and norepinephrine in the brain. As we already know, these brain chemicals assist with attention, reward and motivation. Within this category there are broader groups of medication that may be chosen:

Methylphenidate-based
- Brands: Concerta XL, Ritalin, Equasym XL

- Short-acting or long-acting options
- These are often better tolerated by those who are anxious

Lisdexamfetamine / Dexamfetamine

- Brands: Elvanse (long-acting), Dexedrine (short-acting)
- Often helpful for people with emotional dysregulation or binge-eating patterns
- May be a better fit for those who found methylphenidate unhelpful or mood-flattening
- Tend to have stronger and longer-lasting effects on dopamine and noradrenaline signalling for some

Non-Stimulants (usually second-line or for those who can't tolerate stimulants)

Atomoxetine (brand name Strattera)

- Increases norepinephrine but not a stimulant
- Slower onset; may take 4–6 weeks to feel full effects
- Less risk of abuse or dependence
- Sometimes helpful for ADHD with coexisting anxiety

Guanfacine (Intuniv)

- Affects the prefrontal cortex, useful for hyperactivity or emotional regulation
- Can cause drowsiness or low blood pressure
- Used more often in children but occasionally prescribed off-label in adults

Accessing medication

If you are suitable and want medication for your ADHD, the next challenge can be accessing it. The initial assessment of suitability should be done by your ADHD specialist. They should discuss with you the goals and expectations of treatment and any potential side effects and risks to look out for. They will most likely check some vital statistics such as your pulse rate, blood pressure and weight and they should start the initial prescription and review you until you are stable. The dose usually starts low and is increased slowly with regular checks for any issues or changes. At this point, most ADHD specialists will want to hand over prescribing to your GP under what is known as a 'shared care agreement'.

Shared care agreements

You can find more detail about shared care agreements in Chapter 5, but here's quick summary: shared care agreements are formal arrangements between specialists and GPs to share responsibility for a patient's treatment, usually in conditions requiring specialised medication and ongoing monitoring, such as ADHD, rheumatoid arthritis and IBD. The drugs involved must be started and stabilised by a specialist. Frustratingly for many of you with ADHD, GPs are not obligated to take on shared care arrangements. While I understand this can be upsetting for patients, it is often for safety reasons or concerns from the GP about lack of support or experience around the condition or treatment.

ADHD medication will help some of you, but I feel I'd be doing you a disservice if I didn't ask you to think carefully about what this means. What would success look like to you? Success with medication is not going to render you neurotypical. It will not lead to 100 per cent focus or zero distractions. It should mean more mental clarity, less overwhelm, less inattention and more emotional regulation. Remember, not everyone can do all these things all the time. My final word of caution when it comes to medication for ADHD is to consider it as just one part of your journey. Hormonal input, lifestyle interventions and other supports mentioned throughout this book can potentially have just as much impact.

Cognitive shifts in ADHD and perimenopause: what's happening and how to cope

Cognitive shifts refer to fluctuations in brain function, especially in executive functions like attention, working memory, task starting and completion, and brain fog.

These shifts can occur hourly, daily (some days may be better or worse than others), or cyclically linked to hormone changes, stress, overwhelm, and life stage such as perimenopause.

ADHD in perimenopause is a perfect storm of increasing dopamine dysfunction, increasing emotional dysregulation, poorer sleep and stress in midlife, executive function fatigue, brain fog and burnout. Total system overload. Total shutdown.

Types of Cognitive ADHD Shifts

Type of Shift	Description	Example
Fog	Sluggish, unclear thinking, forgetful	'I walk into a room and forget why I'm there'
Hyperfocus	Overly narrow attention on one task, losing track of time	'I planned to check one email and lost three hours'
Flip-flop	Jumping between tasks, hard to sustain attention	'Started cleaning, ended up organising photos, forgot dinner'
Freeze	Inability to start even simple tasks	'I know what to do, but I just can't begin'
Scatter	Disorganised thoughts, overwhelmed by choices	'Too many tabs open – in my brain . . .'

How to cope with ADHD cognitive shifts in perimenopause

Work with the Shifts, Not Against Them

Track your mental energy; become more aware of when your best times to do certain tasks may be and work to that as much as possible. Equally if there are less productive times, avoid these or choose low-demand tasks.

Time and Task Anchoring

Tie tasks to existing routines, known as the 'time anchoring' technique. Take something you do every day at a set time, like brushing your teeth, and tag a task on.

Create 'start rituals' to help with brain-shifting; for example, drink water and light a candle to start your laptop work. Train your brain to rhythm and routine. It's not easy but over time you should find it gets easier.

Chunk and Externalise

Don't rely on working memory; you are not in an exam. Write things down. Use visuals if this helps you: Post-it notes, planners, task jars (e.g. '2-min tasks', 'needs thinking', 'needs phone'). Chunk tasks into micro-steps and break things down. This is not you failing, this is you learning how your brain works and going with it.

Regulate Before You Execute

Note the nervous system soothing tips on page 72. Learn to recognise when you are struggling, when you are feeling over-whelmed and when this is limiting your ability to start a task or switch to a task. Use the soothing strategies, refocus and start again.

Journalling on Your Journey

Some of you may love it, some of you may hate it, but I encourage all of you to give it a go in this context. Women have grown to love it as part of getting to know themselves again with the newfound knowledge they have acquired. Only when we truly know ourselves can we expect others to know us. Here are some prompts and suggestions to jot down that may help you make sense of things.

Top Tip: If you struggle with writing, make voice notes or draw instead.

Making sense of the shifts

- In what ways have I noticed my focus, memory, or emotional regulation changing lately?
- Are there tasks or responsibilities I used to manage better than I do now?
- What patterns have I noticed in my energy, mood, or motivation across my cycle or the month?
- When do I feel most like *myself*?

Prompt: *'My brain used to _____, but now it often _____. I'm learning to adapt by _____.'*

How does overwhelm show up for you?

- What makes me feel overwhelmed?
- What makes me feel less overwhelmed?
- Who makes me feel overwhelmed?
- How does it show up; what happens?
- How do others see me when I'm overwhelmed?

Prompt: *'When I feel overwhelmed, my go-to response is ___. I'd like to try ___ instead.'*

How do my hormones affect my ADHD symptoms?
Many women experience dips in focus, patience, mood or motivation tied to their menstrual cycle.

- Are there days or times in the month when everything feels harder?
- Have I noticed changes in my ADHD symptoms since perimenopause?
- Would tracking my cycles and periods help me understand how my hormones affect my ADHD?

Prompt: *'During the ___ phase of my cycle, I notice ___. I can prepare by ___.'*

What supportive strategies help me most?

- What helps me get started on hard tasks (e.g. music, body-doubling, timers)?
- What routines help me feel safe and secure right now?
- Where could I introduce more visual or sensory cues to help with memory and motivation?

Prompt: *'One routine that really helps me is ___. I want to now try this in ___.'*

Where am I still masking and what do I need to stop? How can I do this?

- In which areas of my life am I still 'holding it together' at a cost to myself?
- Where do I feel safe enough to be real about how my brain works?

- Who do I feel safe with?
- What boundaries do I need to set to drop the mask?

Prompt: *'I'm tired of pretending ___. I'm ready to ask for ___.'*

What would it look like to lead with self-compassion?

- What would I say to a friend going through what I'm feeling?
- How can I talk to myself differently in hard moments?
- Where can I replace judgement with curiosity?
- Who or what doesn't allow me to do this in my life?
- Can this change and how?

Prompt: *'I'm not failing. I'm adjusting. I am learning to ___, and that's enough for today.'*

Who do I want to be?
This isn't the end of your ability to be who you want to be. It is the beginning of owning who you are and getting the most from it.

Prompt: *'The version of me I'm becoming is ___. I will nurture her by ___.'*

Finally, as I have said before, put positive affirmations in your wallet, your fridge, your mirror, your car, wherever you can. Find your own, but here are some examples:

- ✓ Overwhelm is not a failure, it's a sign to reboot
- ✓ Rest is a necessity not a luxury
- ✓ My brain works well, just at my pace on my terms
- ✓ I am not failing. I am building a life that fits me

It's time to start rewriting your inner voice, believing in yourself and smashing life.

I hope as we head towards the last chapter you are starting to feel more confident in your journey of self-discovery and empowered to move forwards to a more fulfilled and confident self. In the final chapter I will share my tips on how to cocoon yourself in love and support to thrive as your new self.

TL;DR – Chapter 7 Hormones, HRT, ADHD Medication and Cognition Support

Hormone Replacement Therapy (HRT)

- **Forms of HRT**: Tablets, patches, gels, or sprays – choice depends on personal preference and medical history.
- **Progesterone in HRT**: Most women need both oestrogen and progesterone (combined HRT) for womb protection. Some women, especially post-hysterectomy, can take oestrogen-only HRT. If you are perimenopausal you will have progesterone part of the month (sequential regime) and if menopausal all of the month (continuous regime).
- **Transdermal HRT** (patch/gel/spray) is preferred over oral HRT in many women, as it avoids the liver, reducing risks of blood clots and stroke.
- **Different types of progesterone:**
  - **Micronised progesterone** (body-identical) is more natural (chemically identical to the progesterone your body produces) and better tolerated than synthetic progestins by most women, but this is not a given.
  - Responses to progestogens can vary greatly based on genetics, hormone receptor sensitivity, route of administration, and other factors.

- **Challenges with HRT for ADHD:**
  - There is **no one-size-fits-all** approach to HRT, especially for ADHD. Some women may struggle with the progestogen element of HRT, which can lead to side effects like anxiety, mood swings, or bloating.
  - **Lack of research:** There are no gold-standard trials specifically on HRT's effects on ADHD. Most evidence is anecdotal.
  - **HRT and ADHD medication:** Stimulants for ADHD (e.g. methylphenidate) could theoretically interact with HRT, particularly concerning cardio-vascular risks.

- **Progestogen sensitivity:**
  - **Genetic differences, liver function,** and **psycho-logical factors** can affect how a woman responds to progestogen.
  - **Progesterone intolerance** is common, and some women may not tolerate certain progestogens well, leading to discontinuation of HRT.
  - Women with ADHD may benefit from **HRT**, especially in terms of cognition, mood and attention, but there's no definitive answer yet on which HRT type or route works best for ADHD.
  - Women with ADHD should **advocate for themselves** if they don't tolerate a progestogen and work with their GP to adjust dose, route or type.

- **Research gaps:**
  - We need **randomised controlled trials (RCTs)** to better understand the interaction between ADHD, HRT, and long-term health outcomes.
  - Exploration is needed into the **effects of different progestogens** on dopamine regulation in ADHD.

- **What you can do:**
  - Feel empowered to **seek support** from your GP or specialist to find the right HRT regimen for you.
  - Be proactive in discussing potential **side effects** and ask for adjustments if needed.
  - Monitor your response over time, as **HRT is a journey**, not a quick fix.

Nutrition and lifestyle

- **Omega-3 fatty acids**
  - **EPA > DHA:** EPA is best for ADHD (improves attention, mood).
  - **Food sources:** Mackerel, salmon, walnuts (ALA).
  - **Dosage:** 500–1,000mg EPA daily, higher EPA-to-DHA ratio.

- **Other nutrients**
  - **Iron, zinc, magnesium, vitamin D:** Often low in ADHD, supplementation helps brain function.
  - **Avoid:** Alcohol, excess caffeine, sugar, ultra-processed foods.

- **Exercise**
  - Supports dopamine, norepinephrine and serotonin; improves mood, attention and impulse control.
  - **30 mins/day** and strength training 2x/week.

- **Sleep:** ADHD and perimenopause disrupt sleep; good sleep hygiene is crucial.

- **Mindfulness and stress reduction**
  - Reduces emotional reactivity, improves attention.
  - Start with 1–3 minutes of meditation or deep breathing.

- **Structure and environment:** Use planners, timers, and declutter to reduce decision fatigue.

ADHD medication

- **Stimulants**: Methylphenidate (Concerta, Ritalin), Lisdexamfetamine (Elvanse).
- **Non-Stimulants**: Atomoxetine (Strattera), Guanfacine (Intuniv).
- **Access**: Requires ADHD specialist assessment and may involve GP under 'shared care'.

Cognitive shifts

- Common types of shifts in ADHD and perimenopause:
  - **Fog**: Sluggish thinking, forgetfulness.
  - **Hyperfocus**: Too narrow attention, losing track of time.
  - **Flip-flop**: Switching tasks, hard to focus.
  - **Freeze**: Unable to start tasks.
  - **Scatter**: Disorganised thoughts, overwhelmed by choices.

Strategies for coping with cognitive shifts:

- Plan your day around mental energy levels and (un)productive times
- Use time and task anchoring to help start and switch tasks
- Break things down and externalise using tools
- Soothe and regulate your nervous system before executing tasks
- Try journalling to make sense of your journey

Chapter 8
Building Your Support System

Topics covered in this chapter:

- Believing you deserve support: challenging the myth of ADHD over-diagnosis
- ADHD in midlife: how to build a support system with your GP after diagnosis
- ADHD-friendly strategies at home and work: how to find success and support in your workplace and your relationships
- Community, peer support and online spaces

Most of the midlife women I hear from, diagnosed or self-identifying with ADHD later in life, are not only fighting an outward battle but also an internal one with their learned inner voice (see Chapter 6). So many of you don't even want to tell loved ones, let alone medical professionals, about your ADHD for fear of being disbelieved or dismissed. You may feel a long way from asking for support. In my experience, many younger women in their 40s also feel this way about seeking support for perimenopause and together it can all seem just too much to handle.

If this sounds familiar, I want to use this final chapter to give you the conviction that you deserve a support system, and the tools to build one for yourself. I want to arm you with the courage to challenge dismissal, disbelief and in some cases ridicule. Until you truly believe you deserve support, you will not build it around yourself successfully. In fact, you don't just deserve support – you have a right to it, and so do our daughters and granddaughters. I believe you are not just fighting this battle for yourself; you are doing it for every woman before and after you.

We will look at how you can partner with your GP or healthcare team to get the support you need, exploring what helps and what may hinder your care. I will provide some toolbox tips for how to get the most support from your relationships and the workplace, notwithstanding the challenges you may face with both perimenopause and ADHD. Finally, we will also cover how you can access community, peer and online spaces to maximise your potential and inner peace.

Believing you deserve support: challenging the view of ADHD over-diagnosis

There has been a noticeable surge in conversations about ADHD and perimenopause recently, particularly among women in their 30s, 40s and 50s. Social media, podcasts, books, online forums and growing clinic waiting lists reflect the increase in these discussions. If you have read the rest of this book, you'll have a good sense of the complexities around this phenomenon. For some, including clinicians, this tidal wave of awareness causes them to challenge its authenticity; a GP colleague asked me recently 'why does everyone suddenly think they have ADHD or hormone issues?'

The reality, I believe, is rooted in years upon years of under-recognition and underfunding in almost any health condition that predominantly affects women, alongside gender bias towards men and their health needs, and a growing understanding of neurodivergence and women's health. Here are some key arguments to put in your toolbox, because we shouldn't let this go unchallenged if we want things to change for the better.

1. **Delayed recognition is not the same as sudden over-diagnosis**

   For most midlife women, ADHD symptoms will have been present in childhood. Unfortunately, they were also likely successfully masked and missed by everyone around them. It is now well known that girls with ADHD often go unnoticed because they are far less likely to present as hyperactive or disruptive. Instead, these are the girls described as daydreamers, perfectionists, anxious or never quite meeting their potential. In later life they may be described as 'dizzy' or 'ditsy'. This is not women suddenly hitting midlife and deciding they want to rewrite their story; this is a travesty of the highest order.

   Likewise, perimenopause and menopause have forever been discussed primarily in terms of hot flushes and periods stopping, yet for many, the most distressing symptoms are psychological or cognitive decline: mood swings, brain fog, irritability, exhaustion. Not to mention many other unrecognised physical symptoms such as aches and pains, insomnia and palpitations. These too have often been dismissed, misdiagnosed as depression or fibromyalgia, or put down to stress. Recognising them now doesn't mean women are finding these problems earlier, it means we didn't support them to be recognised sooner.

2. **We have started to listen more to women**

   We're getting better at recognising and listening to women's lived experiences (albeit still with a long way to go). Women continue to push for a voice and as they do this in an age of social media and digitalisation, it picks up pace and knowledge, and empowerment grows. You finally have frameworks to understand what once felt like personal failings: 'Why can't I keep up?' 'Why do I feel like I'm falling apart?' 'Why can I cope one week and not the next?' When you start to recognise these things in yourself, perhaps through diagnosis of your children, exposure to podcasts, or online resources, you may feel seen for the first time. This isn't a case of self-diagnosis gone wild. It's often a long, painful process of making sense of years of struggling to keep up and feel truly capable. We should be apologising to you for years of missed opportunities, not berating you for taking so long to understand yourself. Make sure you remember that.

3. **The overlap is real and sadly understudied**
   There is growing research into and recognition of how hormones impact ADHD in women, specifically with regards to perimenopause. It is basic neuroscience, but it has taken us a long time to start exploring this thoroughly. The rise in conversations around perimenopause and menopause in recent years has naturally led to exploration of other effects that fluctuating hormones can have on women's health and wellbeing. This isn't sudden; it is acceptance of a biologically plausible, clinically relevant relationship that has only recently started to receive the research, attention and discussion it deserves. We aren't there yet but together, we can get there.

4. **Awareness isn't the same as over-diagnosis**
   It's all too easy to dismiss women for health-seeking behaviours that seem new, evolving or leave us wondering what to do. Doing so can minimise the real distress that drives people to seek answers. In my experience, when a midlife woman gets to the

point of seeking help for unravelling, she has hit desperation and needs understanding, validation and support. Increased diagnosis is not always a sign of over-diagnosis; it can be a sign of years of underdiagnosis preceding it.

5. **Does anyone truly want to feel like this?**
Back to the original question from my colleague: why does everyone suddenly think they have ADHD or hormone issues? They don't. It isn't sudden and it isn't wanted. Being perimenopausal doesn't suddenly give you the drive to look for problems, it topples your 'just about coping' brain chemistry into chaos. In the process, it unmasks a lifelong neurodevelopmental condition. No woman or man I have ever met in my career as a doctor has chosen to have ADHD, or the challenges that come with living with it in a world that doesn't always understand ADHD. Many have become unique and resilient as a result.

ADHD in midlife: how to build a support system with your GP after diagnosis

Receiving an ADHD diagnosis in your 40s or 50s can offer a complex mix of relief and overwhelm. You finally have an explanation for things that never made sense, the recurrent exhaustion with simple day-to-day existence, the memory lapses and numerous lost keys, the uncontrollable emotional rollercoasters, the burnout. Then you may start to feel that diagnosis is just the start of a whole new chapter of self-discovery, acceptance and fulfilment.

Now is the time to start creating a support system that helps you to thrive, not just survive with ADHD. This can be especially important as you transition into the menopause alongside the demands of midlife, hormonal changes, family, relationships and careers.

Partnering with a GP or healthcare team that you feel comfortable with and trust after diagnosis can be almost as challenging as getting diagnosed in the first place. If you can do this though, it can also be a game-changer for your onwards journey. There are some key steps I suggest you try and work through to ensure you get the support you need.

1. **Agree on a follow-up plan; don't let it end at diagnosis**
    As a GP I know this one isn't an easy ask for most. Getting appointments with the same GP on a regular basis can be a challenge. For most practices, this will be because of day-to-day changes in GP availability across a week and on-the-day demand for urgent appointments. Most practices will be able to offer review appointments with the same GP on an infrequent basis, perhaps twice a year, so do ask if this is possible. While most practices struggle to provide continuity of care for all patients on a regular basis these days, due to limited resources and changing workforce modelling, we do know that continuity of care has better outcomes for our patients and research backs this. Most GPs want to see their own patients again; it's why many of us became GPs. If you do manage to secure this, these are the things I suggest you cover:

    - How your symptoms are responding to any treatment (medication or otherwise)
    - Any side effects or changes in functioning
    - New challenges that arise as life circumstances evolve

    In my experience, even knowing you have a review appointment scheduled, however far away, can be really comforting to patients.

2. **If you're on medication, get to know your shared care plan**

   If your GP has agreed to a shared care agreement to prescribe for you, I'd recommend taking an interest in what this means for you both. I explain shared care agreements in Chapter 5 – and what to do if your GP hasn't agreed to one – but I recommend also asking your GP to explain how shared care works and, most importantly, what your plan involves. Your agreement likely requests that your GP practice monitor your blood pressure, heart rate, weight and sleep, especially during the first few months of treatment. It is important you attend for these check-ups when asked so they can continue to prescribe safely.

3. **Review hormonal and general health, especially if you're perimenopausal**

   As we've discovered time and time again throughout this book, midlife ADHD comes with its own unique challenges in women. Alongside midlife responsibilities, oestrogen fluctuations can worsen ADHD symptoms significantly.

   Ask your GP about HRT if it is something you feel able to consider. It may also be worth considering possible deficiencies that can cause brain fog, tiredness and further overlapping symptoms such as low iron, B12 and an underactive thyroid. Discuss this with your GP too and see what they think.

   Managing both elements together rather than focusing on one creates a complete picture of your overall health. Look at the lifestyle and holistic toolkit in Chapter 4; these things can really start to make a difference, whatever stage of your journey you are at. It will really show your healthcare team you are taking a teamwork approach and hopefully boost engagement.

4. **Ask about non-medication support**
   There's more to ADHD care than prescriptions. Ask your GP or healthcare team about:

- Occupational therapy for executive function differences (organisation, planning, sensory regulation). This can be limited on the NHS but will vary from area to area.
- ADHD coaching. This is also unlikely to be available on the NHS, but your healthcare team may know of local coaches or groups you can have a chat with for advice about what they may offer and any associated costs.
- ADHD-aware counselling or coaching (sometimes available via Improving Access to Psychological Therapies (IAPT) services or local services).
- Workplace support. You may be entitled to reasonable adjustments or an Access to Work grant. Your GP may not be up to speed on this but should be able to help you by supplying information about your diagnosis to organisations or services that require it, with your permission. They may have access to a social prescriber that can offer support.
- Local or online peer support groups. These can be vital for normalising your experience and picking up practical tips and local intel. Don't wait for a formal diagnosis to access this.

5. **Talk about mental and physical self-care**
   We've explored how many women with ADHD burn out over years of masking, perfectionism and pushing through. Now is the time to recognise that this is not a failing in you. Discuss your mental health with your GP if needed. Having ADHD or perimenopause does not exclude you from having depression, anxiety and other mental health conditions. It does

not make any of these things less valid, but it does make them harder to manage. If you're struggling to prioritise your own care, say so. ADHD often interferes with self-compassion and consistency and knowing this can really help your GP or healthcare team to support you to break this cycle.

6. **Make your support system visible to all parties (including yourself)**
You may be juggling different aspects of support (GP, psychiatry, menopause clinic, therapist, coach, occupational therapy). Consider keeping a written summary of who's doing what and giving consent for different providers to communicate with each other where helpful, so everyone stays on the same page. Not only does this make life easier, but it also makes care less duplicative and more tailored to you.

7. **Speak up about what's not working**
As a GP I rarely get upset about what a patient queries or asks for, even if I'm unable to provide it or think it's not reasonable or sensible. The upset or grumpiness patients may perceive from their GP, healthcare team or practice staff is almost always to do with the manner in which a patient's requests have been addressed.

Over the years, NHS resources have become increasingly stretched and as a result, patients and staff have become increasingly frustrated. This often shows up as anger, rudeness, aggression and escalation from either party. Most of the complaints we receive as a practice stem from poor communication. I totally get how difficult access to timely GP care can be. Despite being a GP myself, I am a patient who must also access other GP services for myself and my family. I've had good and not so good experiences, and I've waited longer than I should have at times. None of us want it to be this way.

If you address things in an understanding and productive way, whether it's medication side effects, HRT making things worse, or difficulty accessing services, you are far more likely to get a more positive response. I know this isn't always the case, and I am not here to excuse poor, unsympathetic care, I'm hoping to make the chances of you getting the opposite of this more successful. People's needs change over time; you shouldn't feel afraid to bring this up. You're not being difficult. You're being proactive and that's exactly what managing a long-term condition requires.

Living well with ADHD in midlife is about creating a network of care and support. There is no single quick fix, including medication. Taking the time and effort to find and build a good relationship with your GP or a trusted clinician if at all possible, can be key.

Getting the best support from your workplace with ADHD

I truly believe there is no limit to what you can achieve as a woman with ADHD, even if you've spent most of your life undiagnosed and unsupported. Women are a resilient and formidable species. When it comes to the workplace, however, some jobs may play to your strengths more than others. You may have already gravitated to some of these roles, or you may feel it's too late in the day to do so, but it can be helpful to stop and take stock through your new lens. Of course, everyone is unique but there are key strengths women with ADHD have often developed (sometimes out of necessity). See if you recognise any of these strengths below:

Core strengths common in women with ADHD

1. **Creativity and Idea Generation**

- Strong ability to think outside the box, connect different dots, and see possibilities others may overlook.
- Comfort with uncertainty, spontaneity and 'blue-sky thinking'.

2. **High Energy and Passion**

- When engaged in something interesting, can work with intense focus and enthusiasm (hyperfocus).
- Brings infectious motivation and enthusiasm to projects.

3. **Strong People Skills, Empathy and Intuition**

- Many women with ADHD are highly attuned to emotions and social cues, often assisted by years of masking.
- Ability to build rapport quickly and read between the lines.

4. **Adaptability and Problem-Solving**

- Can pivot quickly when plans change.
- Often resourceful in finding unconventional solutions.

5. **Risk-Taking and Innovation**

- Willing to try new approaches and challenge the status quo.
- Can often spot opportunities others miss.

6. **Multitasking Under Pressure**
- Despite the obvious issue with task starting and switching, once engaged and focused, can often flip

and juggle multiple priorities in fast-moving environments (though repetitive, slow-paced tasks may drain energy).

7. **Storytelling and Communication**
   - Many have strong verbal expression, humour, or narrative skills, making them engaging presenters or communicators.

ADHD brains thrive when there is variety, innovation and depth of meaning to a role. For these reasons, you may find you excel in roles that are mission-driven, fast-paced, creative or caring. The options are endless: design, nursing, entrepreneurial, event planning, product development, charity work and many more sectors can all be rewarding. Repetitive, detail-heavy and rigidly structured roles without flexibility or innovation and change can be draining unless there's strong support or systems in place. By the time you land here, reading this book, you are likely also perimenopausal and to some degree feeling quite fraught at work or even experiencing burnout (more about this further down and in Chapter 3).

In an ideal world you would be in a supportive work environment that plays to your strengths and skills. In the real world this may not be the case, although many workplaces are slowly starting to look with supportive curiosity at neurodivergence in the workplace. Here are my tips to seek that support:

Get clear on your needs first, considering these alone or with a supportive colleague:

- Think about specific situations where ADHD or perimenopause make work harder (e.g. noisy environments, memory, organisation, fatigue, hot flushes, anxiety before meetings).
- Translate them into practical supports (e.g. quiet

workspace, flexibility with deadlines, written instructions, regular breaks, temperature control).

Reasonable adjustment examples to consider:

- Extended deadlines
- Regular short manager check-ins to review priorities and asks
- Flexible hours
- Written asks over verbal ones
- A headset for meetings or noise-cancelling headphones for the office
- Clear task priorities
- Low-distraction workspace
- Meetings recorded
- Airy rooms that can have opening windows and/or air conditioning
- Protected conversation: You're entitled to raise these needs without fear of dismissal or harassment.

Employers may refer you to Occupational Health for assessment to guide adjustments. This is usually a positive step. Some workplaces now have menopause policies and/or neurodiversity policies in place, so it's worth checking if this is the case too.

Here's an example of how to present your request:

'These are some adjustments that would help me manage my health conditions and work at my best. They are considered reasonable under UK workplace law, and many are simple, low-cost changes.'

Know your rights; your employer may have a legal duty to make reasonable adjustments.

It's always better to have an open and honest conversation with your line manager or employer first; hopefully they will want to support you to get the best work from you and keep you well. Sometimes, you may need to know your rights if things don't go to plan and there is some legal support in the UK as outlined below.

- **Equality Act 2010**
  Protects against discrimination at work. Applies if you have a 'disability' which is defined as a physical or mental impairment that has a substantial and long-term adverse effect on your ability to carry out normal day-to-day activities. ADHD often (not always) meets this definition, especially if symptoms significantly impact daily functioning. Perimenopause is not automatically a disability, but if symptoms (e.g. brain fog, fatigue, anxiety, hot flushes) are severe and long-lasting, they can fall under this definition too.

- **Health and Safety at Work Act 1974**
  Employers must ensure the health, safety and welfare of employees. For perimenopause, this can include temperature control, uniform adaptations, and ventilation. For ADHD, it can include environmental adjustments (quiet spaces, reduced distractions), workload structuring and clarity in communication.

- **Employment Rights Act 1996**
  Protects against unfair dismissal. If someone is dismissed or treated unfairly due to ADHD or menopause symptoms (without support being considered), that *may* count as discrimination or unfair dismissal.

- **Case Law**
  Tribunals have already ruled that menopause symptoms can amount to a disability under the Equality Act (e.g. Davies v Scottish Courts

and Tribunals Service). ADHD is increasingly recognised as a neurodivergence requiring adjustments.

Frame the conversation around performance and solutions:

- Position it as: 'These changes would help me work at my best and continue contributing fully.'
- Employers are likely to respond better when you're proactive and collaborative.

Decide how much to disclose:

You don't have to give every detail. Some people simply say: 'I'm managing health conditions that affect my concentration/energy at times' and then ask for specific adjustments. Others are open about ADHD and perimenopause if they feel the culture is supportive.

Seek allies:

- HR, Occupational Health, or line managers trained in wellbeing and/or equity, diversity and inclusion (EDI) can be advocates.
- If there's a women's network, neurodiversity network, or union rep – they're valuable allies too.

What to expect

You may find mixed awareness levels. Some managers are well-educated on menopause and/or ADHD, while others may not have a clue. Be prepared to signpost them to resources (these can be found on page 209). Agreed adjustments (e.g. flexible hours, cooling fans, project management tools) may need tweaking. Expect reasonable pushback; employers may weigh up what's 'reasonable' in the context of the role. Workplace conversations around both menopause and neurodiversity are expanding, so you may find more support than you expect.

Why bother 'tackling' the workplace

Unsupported ADHD in perimenopause can lead to poor performance and wellbeing at work. With small adjustments, many of the challenges become manageable, creating a better outcome for you, your colleagues and your employer. Retaining skilled staff is better for employers than losing them. By speaking up, you're also helping to normalise these discussions, paving the way for others.

Mindset and maintenance at work (and outside it)

Be realistic about what you expect of yourself. That's not to say you cannot achieve anything you want to, but you will need to build systems and processes that support you in doing this, not expect you to operate the same way as others who are not living with ADHD and perimenopause. There will be some days that are easier than others. This happens to us all but can be more pronounced if you have ADHD, are perimenopausal or both. Accept these and move forwards, remembering that one bad day or episode does not define who you are and what you are capable of.

- Now may be the time to let go of 'perfect' and aim for sustainable, repeatable and good enough. If you struggle with this concept, consider what or where has striving for perfection got you so far. Was it worth it? Is good enough actually good enough?
- Use rewards and novelty; your brain thrives on dopamine. Find relatively healthy things that will bring you dopamine boosts as rewards for completing tasks.
- Forgive yourself and be compassionate. You are not stupid, overly emotional, lazy or useless. You are working with your brain, not against it.

Remember the routines and rituals that work wherever you are:

- Anchoring: Linking tasks together so they happen on autopilot (e.g. brush teeth → take meds → make bed).
- Visuals: Whiteboards, sticky notes, or app reminders where you see them, not buried in a drawer or under clutter.
- Pre-decide everything: Pick two breakfast options and two sets of work clothes the night before to reduce daily decision fatigue. When you're making these decisions in the moment, they become more pressured.
- Keep a 'brain dump' notebook or use an app for random thoughts and lists so your mind can stop holding everything at once. Overwhelm leads to shutdown, shutdown leads to meltdown. Proactively instigate things that break these destructive cycles.
- Write everything down; lots of people do this for various reasons. Don't be ashamed; normalise it.
- Use digital or tangible timers (e.g. a Time Timer, Pomodoro timer, digital watch, or kitchen timer) to make time visible and thus real to you.
- Set alarms or ask people to 'move you on' between tasks. This can help transitions. If you have a desk job, schedule things like 'drive to next meeting' etc. This can avoid arriving at start times and not being ready to begin. Try to put scaffolding in that prevents you slipping into the 'now and not now' zone of time blindness.
- Try 'parking' unfinished tasks with a note on them detailing what you need to do next. This will make restarting unfinished tasks so much easier.
- Simplify your workspaces or home. Create areas for everything and store things in the room you use

them, not where you might be 'supposed to' store them. Have extras of things like phone chargers, pens, reading specs to lower stress under time pressure when memory falters. Invest in tools like key trackers and 'find my phone' apps.

- Build in breaks, if possible, between tasks and look to anything that can improve your sensory inputs, e.g. noise-cancelling headphones.

How to keep your relationships intact with ADHD and get the support you need

People with ADHD are some of the most caring and empathic people I have met, with a keen sense of intuition, who can be extremely loving parents and partners. However, ADHD traits can also cause some relationship difficulties if not handled well and misunderstood. The effects of your ADHD on your relationships, both romantic and platonic, can be varied and widespread. Here are some of the factors that may play a part in conflict or relationship breakdown:

- Attention (you may tune out unintentionally, seem disinterested, uncaring)
- Memory (you might forget plans, conversations, or birthdays, not deliver an ask)
- Time (you may run late or lose track of tasks, seem unreliable)
- Emotion (you can be quick to react or deeply affected by perceived rejection or criticism, which can seem 'easily triggered' if not understood)
- Initiation (you might struggle to start conversations or follow through)
- Completion (you might not always complete what

is asked of you or follow through, which can lead to
you seeming unreliable or uncommitted)

These may be neurobiological features of your ADHD but
if left unexplained or misunderstood, they can quite quickly
lead to resentment and conflict.

Relationship strategies to build your support

Identify so others can understand and recognise

You don't need to share everything if you prefer not to, but identifying where things may look different to your intention can be
helpful in all kinds of relationships, including your friendships.

Example: 'Sometimes I forget things or interrupt without
meaning to. I'll try not to, but I just wanted to say I know it
can be frustrating. Please don't take it personally.'

Use tools that help you stay reliable and committed

If this fails, be open and honest about why.

Example: 'I know it looks like I don't care when I forget
important things. I do really care but my memory struggles at
times to stay on message.'

Manage emotional reactivity

ADHD often comes with rejection sensitive dysphoria
(extreme reaction to perceived criticism or rejection), impulsive responses, justice sensitivity (which we mentioned briefly
on page 64) or emotional outbursts. This can be particularly
damaging in relationships, including parenting. Being perimenopausal or menopausal will likely exacerbate this.

Having ADHD or hormonal changes may make this reactivity trickier to handle but it should never be an excuse for

acceptance of poor behaviour towards others. Owning your behaviours and taking accountability, alongside discussing with your partner, relative or friend how you can work together to manage this can be a game-changer for everyone.

Examples: 'I feel overwhelmed when plans change last-minute. Can we try to stick to plans where possible or if not, can you give me as much notice as possible please?'

'I'm sorry I overreacted. When you said this x, I felt that y. My response was uncalled for; can we please talk about it and try again?'

'I'm feeling overwhelmed right now so I'm going to take a few minutes before I respond – don't think I'm snubbing you.'

Modelling this behaviour of ownership, accountability and open communication can be great for children to develop too.

Talk about roles and expectations

In longer term relationships with partners or even in parent–child relationships and friendships, one person can become the 'manager' and the other the 'managed'. The manager will take on the mental load of planning, organising, running the finances and home and whatever else keeps life ticking over. If this is mutually agreed and accepted, things will go better than if roles are assumed and in turn feel unbalanced. In ADHD, this imbalance can be easy to fall into without pre-planning and open discussion. Combat this by being open and honest about who does what and why this works for both of you (or not).

Communicate more than you think you should (it's probably still not enough)

You may be prone to assuming others know what you mean or think. Communicate, confirm and clarify at all points. Name your thoughts and emotions so others are clear, if you are prone to being misunderstood. Express what you need to feel safe and perform well.

Examples: 'I'm not upset, I'm just distracted and need to focus on this for 10 minutes.'

'I really value how you remind me without judging.'

Repair and reconnect

Don't use ADHD as an excuse for poor behaviour. Apologise, aim to do better, take accountability. Take regular intervals to spend z time with your partner, child or loved ones. Sometimes you may seem preoccupied, stressed or 'all over the place'. Taking time out and investing in relationships is a good piece of self-care. If you have people around you who truly support you, this is some of the best scaffolding you can have.

Connect others with support

Encourage partners and/or close family members to:

- Learn about ADHD through books (*ADHD 2.0: New Science and Essential Strategies*; *Dirty Laundry: Why Adults with ADHD Are So Ashamed and What We Can Do to Help*; *Your Brain's Not Broken: Strategies for Navigating Your Emotions and Life with ADHD* are good places to start)
- Join support groups for partners of those with ADHD
- Be open to relationship coaching or counselling; especially if burnout or communication breakdowns are present

Community, peer support and online spaces

Medical care, like medication and ADHD clinics, can only offer part of the solution to living well with ADHD and perimenopause. Throughout this book, you've also learned about other things that can help you thrive rather than survive, including lifestyle changes, new rituals and routines. Building a meaningful ADHD support community through peers and online can also be a valuable part of your journey. Thousands of women just like you know exactly how you feel or have felt; you just need to find them. It goes without saying you also know just how other women with ADHD and perimenopause will be feeling or have felt and you can help each other feel less alone and more validated, as well as sharing practical tips on how to thrive. Go to page 209 for a valuable bank of resources you can access.

Be wary of becoming overloaded. Take it in small manageable chunks and ask others you meet for recommendations of what resources have helped them feel supported. Choose groups that feel supportive, not overwhelming. Set your boundaries and don't stay if somewhere isn't beneficial for you.

ADHD in midlife may be very personal, but it's also a shared experience and story for many other women too. Build a community that can offer you not just practical help but also hope and a sense of belonging. Don't underestimate it. Feeling seen, heard and truly understood should not be a luxury you can do without. I consider it a necessity for you to move forwards on this journey.

TL;DR – Chapter 8: Building Your Support System

Believing you deserve support

- Internal struggle with feeling undeserving of support due to fear of dismissal.
- Support is essential, not just for you but for future generations.

Why ADHD and perimenopause are 'suddenly' a thing

- **Delayed recognition**: ADHD symptoms often masked in childhood, perimenopause symptoms misdiagnosed.
- **Women's voices**: Better recognition of women's health experiences, particularly with ADHD and hormonal changes.
- **Hormonal impact**: Growing research on how hormones affect ADHD in women.
- **Increased diagnosis**: A surge in diagnoses isn't over-diagnosis; it's addressing years of underdiagnosis.
- **No one wants this**: ADHD and perimenopause isn't something women 'choose' to have, it's often a result of accumulated struggles.

Partnering with your GP for ADHD care

Follow-up plan: Schedule regular check-ins to monitor medication and treatment progress.

Shared care plan: Understand your medication management plan, including health checks (blood pressure, sleep, etc.).

Review hormonal and general health: Address hormonal fluctuations and other health issues like iron/B12 deficiencies or thyroid issues.

Non-medication support: Explore options like ADHD coaching, occupational therapy, workplace accommodations, and mental health care.

Self-care: Discuss mental and physical wellbeing and ask for support with self-compassion and consistency.

Visibility of your support system: Keep a summary of all healthcare providers and communication to ensure coordinated care.

Speak up about what's not working: Proactively address concerns with your healthcare team; clear communication leads to better outcomes.

The bigger picture: ADHD in midlife is about more than just medication; building a strong, supportive network is crucial for thriving through ADHD and perimenopause.

Getting support at work

- Play to your strengths: ADHD women are often creative, empathetic, adaptable, intuitive, high-energy, great problem-solvers.
- Identify challenges (e.g. distractions, memory, fatigue).
- Ask for *reasonable adjustments* like:
    - Flexible hours/deadlines
    - Noise-cancelling headphones
    - Clear task lists
    - Quiet or cool workspace

Know your rights (UK):

- **Equality Act 2010** – ADHD often counts as a disability.
- Menopause symptoms may qualify too.
- Employers must make *reasonable adjustments* where the Equality Act applies.

How to ask:

- Frame it as: 'These changes help me perform at my best.'
- Disclose only what you're comfortable with.

- HR, Occupational Health and networks can support.

Mindset tips:

- Let go of perfection – aim for *good enough*.
- Use lists, timers, reminders and visual cues.
- Build breaks into your day and simplify your space.

Relationships:

- Be honest about your ADHD traits.
- Take responsibility, communicate clearly, and repair conflicts when needed.

Find community:

- Join peer/online support groups.
- Share, learn and feel less alone.

With understanding, small adjustments and the right support, you can thrive at work and at home.

Closing remarks

As we bring this final chapter to a close, I hope you feel in a better position to move forwards on your journey towards your authentic self. You've travelled a long way through these pages. You may have recognised yourself in the stories of ADHD and perimenopause, found language for the burnout you've been carrying, or discovered why masking has been so exhausting for so long. Perhaps you've even taken some first steps towards diagnosis, self-identification, or simply allowing yourself to be you without apology.

Wherever you are right now, know this: you have already done something powerful. You've given yourself the gift of awareness.

This book was never meant to be just information; it was meant to be a companion. Something to lean on when your focus slips, when your energy dips, or when the world feels too loud or against you. It was written to remind you that you are not alone, that what you are experiencing is real, and that there is a way forward that honours who you are.

The truth is that midlife is not an ending. It is a recalibration. For many of us, it's the first time we stop living by everyone else's expectations and start asking: what do I need, what do I want, and how do I thrive from here? It's not always about rediscovering who you were; it's deciding who you are now and being your best self.

What comes next?

- Keep using the toolkits and resources in this book as often as you need them. They are here to support you, not just once, but on repeat.
- Share what you've learned. Talking openly about ADHD and perimenopause to help dismantle the silence and stigma can not only change your life, but it can also be life-changing for others walking a similar path.
- Celebrate your strengths. Your creativity, empathy, energy and resilience are not accidents, they are you.

And finally...

This journey is not about becoming someone new. It's about uncovering the person you've always been beneath the layers of coping, masking and pushing through. Your journey doesn't end here. In fact, it begins here: with clarity, compassion, and the courage to live unapologetically as yourself.

Remember, you are always believed here.

The time is now. And you are ready.

Resources

PODCASTS AND VIDEOS

ADHD Chatter, Alex Partridge
ADHD Peri Punks, Chrissy Ingram and Sarah Glasco
Faster Than Normal, Peter Shankman
How To ADHD, Jessica McCabe (YouTube)
The ADHD Adults Podcast, James Brown and Alex Conner
The ADHD Women's Wellbeing Podcast, Kate Moryoussef
The Neurodivergent Woman, Michelle Livock and Monique
    Mitchelson
TEDx Talks – search for 'ADHD in Women' (YouTube/www.
    ted.com)

MAGAZINES AND WEBSITES

ADDISS: National Attention Deficit Disorder Information and
    Support Service (www.addiss.co.uk)
Additude (additudemag.com)
ADHD UK (adhduk.co.uk)
NHS: ADHD in Adults (www.nhs.uk/conditions/adhd-adults)

BOOKS

ADHD 2.0: New Science and Essential Strategies, Edward Hallowell
    and John Ratey
ADHD for Smart Ass Women, Tracy Otsuka
*Allow Me to Interrupt: A psychologist reveals the emotional truth behind
    women's ADHD*, Gilly Kahn
*Dirty Laundry: Why Adults with ADHD Are So Ashamed and What We
    Can Do to Help*, Richard Pink

How To Thrive with Adult ADHD, James Kustlow
It's Not a Bloody Trend: Understanding life as an ADHD adult,
    Kat Brown
*Now It All Makes Sense: How an ADHD Diagnosis Brought Clarity to
    My Life*, Alex Partridge
The ADHD Women's Wellbeing Toolkit, Kate Moryoussef
*Wise Power: Discover the liberating power of menopause to awaken
    authority, purpose and belonging*, Alexandra Pope and Sjanie Hugo
    Wurlitzer
*Your Brain's Not Broken: Strategies for Navigating Your Emotions and
    Life with ADHD*, Tamara Rosier

SUPPORT GROUPS, COACHING
AND WORKSHOPS

ADHDAF+ Charity (www.adhdafplus.org.uk/peersupport)
ADHD Women's Wellbeing by Kate Moryoussef (www.adhdwom-
    enswellbeing.co.uk)
Dr Helen Wall runs information pages on Facebook and Instagram
    (no personal medical advice). This is a peer support/coaching
    community, not medical care. If you're in crisis or feel unsafe, use
    urgent services. While it can be helpful for shared experience and
    strategies, it is not a diagnostic service.

A note for readers: be mindful of validity and accuracy in Instagram
and TikTok content creators and ADHD educators. YouTube is a
great source of bite-sized explainers, lived experiences and strategy
demonstrations.

References

In order of use throughout this book

Attoe, D. E. and Climie, E. A., 'Miss. Diagnosis: A systematic review of ADHD in adult women', *Journal of Attention Disorders*, 27:7 (2023), pp. 645–57

Biederman, J. et al., 'Females with ADHD: An expert consensus statement taking a lifespan approach providing guidance for the identification and treatment of attention-deficit/hyperactivity disorder in girls and women', *BMC Psychiatry*, 20:404 (2020)

Demontis, D., Walters, R. K., Martin, J., et al., 'Discovery of the first genome-wide significant risk loci for attention deficit/hyperactivity disorder', *Nature Genetics*, 51:1 (2019), pp. 63–75

Rommelse, N. N. J., Franke, B., Geurts, H. M., et al., 'Shared heritability of attention-deficit/hyperactivity disorder and autism spectrum disorder', *European Child & Adolescent Psychiatry*, 19:3 (2010), pp. 281–95

Lundström, S., Reichenberg, A., Anckarsäter, H., et al., 'Autism and co-occurring ADHD explained by genetic overlap', *Journal of Child Psychology and Psychiatry*, 53:1 (2012), pp. 126–36

Franke, B. et al., 'The heritability of ADHD in children of ADHD parents: a post hoc analysis of longitudinal data', *Journal of Neurodevelopmental Disorders*, 15:24 (2023)

Faraone, S. V. and Larsson, H., 'Genetics of attention deficit hyperactivity disorder', *Molecular Psychiatry*, 24:4 (2019), pp. 562–75

Kim, C., Asnicar, F., Marples, L., et al., 'Associations between gut microbiota and menopause symptoms: novel insights from the ZOE PREDICT 3 cohort', *Proceedings of the Nutrition Society*, 84(OCE3), E243 (2025)

Shaw, P. et al., 'Attention-deficit/hyperactivity disorder is

characterized by a delay in cortical maturation', *PNAS*, 104:49
(2007), pp. 19649–54

Hoogman, M. et al., 'Subcortical brain volume differences in partici-
pants with ADHD across the lifespan: an ENIGMA collabor-
ation', *The Lancet Psychiatry*, 4:4 (2017), 310–19

Castellanos, F. X. et al., 'Cingulate-Precuneus Interactions: A New
Locus of Dysfunction in Adult ADHD', *Biological Psychiatry*, 63:3
(2008), pp. 332–7

Volkow, N. D. et al., 'Evaluating dopamine reward pathway in ADHD:
clinical implications', *JAMA*, 302:10 (2009), pp. 1084–91

Yu, M., Gao, X., Niu, X., et al., 'Meta analysis of structural and
functional alterations of brain in patients with attention deficit/
hyperactivity disorder', *Frontiers in Psychiatry*, 13, Art, 1070142
(2023)

Smith, S. S. et al., 'Progesterone metabolites regulate GABA-A
receptors', *Annals of the NY Academy of Sciences* (1998)

Petersen, N. et al., 'Estradiol and progesterone influence on
dopamine reward sensitivity', *Psychoneuroendocrinology* (2014)

Office for National Statistics, 'Suicides in the United Kingdom: 2023
data' (2023) [Available online at: www.ons.gov.uk]

Biederman, J., Wilens, T. E. and Faraone, S. V., 'The impact of ADHD
on the risk of suicide in adults: A review of the literature', *Journal
of Attention Disorders*, 26:9 (2022), pp. 1257–66

McDonough, M., and Singh, S., 'Suicide risk in women with ADHD:
Evidence from a national cohort study', *Journal of Clinical
Psychiatry*, 80:5 (2019), pp. 123–30

Hawton, K., and Heeringen, K. V., 'Suicide: An updated review of the
literature', *The Lancet*, 373:9672 (2009), pp. 1372–81

Kuehn, B. M., 'Estrogen and the Brain: The Impact of Estrogen on
Neurotransmitter Systems in Women', *JAMA Psychiatry*, 74:4
(2017), pp. 421–2

Strogatz, S. H. and Kronauer, R. E., 'Understanding the biology of
sleep and circadian rhythms', *Sleep Medicine Reviews*, 6:5 (1989),
pp. 273–83

Faraone, S. V. and Buitelaar, J., 'Comparing the efficacy of stimulants
for ADHD in children and adolescents using meta-analysis',
European Child & Adolescent Psychiatry, 19:4 (2010), pp. 353–64

Acknowledgements

This book would not have been possible without the exceptional team at Penguin. My heartfelt thanks to Anya Hayes, Céline Nyssens and the wider publishing team for your talent, care and unwavering support. Your belief in this work, your insight and your calm guidance have meant more than I can say.

To my GP partners and the entire practice team at The Oaks Family Practice, Bolton: thank you for your constant support, patience and collegiality. Your encouragement has allowed me the space to think, to write and to keep advocating for better care, even on the busiest of days. To my best friend of over 40 years, Alison: forever in my corner. To Linda, for keeping me sane as I find myself.

Most importantly, my deepest thanks go to the women who have come to me as patients and followers and placed your trust in me. You have shared your stories, your struggles and your resilience with honesty and courage. You have taught me more than any textbook ever could. This book exists because of you, and it is my hope that, because of you, many more women will be heard, understood and supported to do better.

Last, but never least, I honour the strong women who shaped me into the woman, mother and doctor I am today. To my mum and my best friend June Wall (Hobson), taken far too soon and missed every single day – this book carries your love and resilience in every page. And to Dr Julie McMillen, an extraordinary GP who was my inspiration, my guide and my constant compass. You were both fierce advocates for women, quietly brave and unwavering in your principles. I miss you beyond words, but I hope this work reflects the values you lived by – and that, in some small way, it would make you proud.